The

BLACK MAN'S GUIDE TO GOOD HEALTH

OTHER BOOKS BY NEIL SHULMAN INCLUDE

Doc Hollywood
Your Body's Red Light Warning System

The
BLACK MAN'S GUIDE TO GOOD HEALTH

ESSENTIAL ADVICE FOR AFRICAN AMERICAN MEN AND THEIR FAMILIES

NEW AND REVISED EDITION

James W. Reed, M. D., F.A.C.P.
Neil Shulman, M.D.,
And Charlene Shucker

HILTON PUBLISHING COMPANY • ROSCOE, ILLINOIS

Published by Hilton Publishing Company
PO Box 737, Roscoe, IL 61073
815-885-1070
www.hiltonpub.com

Publisher's Cataloging-in-Publication
(Provided by Quality Books, Inc.)

Reed, James, 1944–
      The black man's guide to good health : essential advice for the special concerns of African-American men / James W. Reed, Neil B. Shulman, and Charlene Shucker.—2nd rev. ed.
      p. cm.
      Includes bibliographical references.
      ISBN: 0–9675258–1–0

      1. Afro-American men—Health and hygiene. 2. Afro-American men—Diseases. I. Shulman, Neil. II. Shucker, Charlene. III. Title.

RA777.8.R44 2000   616/.04234/08996073
                                     QBI00–541

Printed and bound in the United States of America

I dedicate this book to my sons, David Michael Reed and Robert Anthony Reed, with the wish that this book may help them to live still more happy and productive lives.

—James Reed

I dedicate this book to Israel, Mary, Larry, Stan, Roberta, Andy, Jon, Josh, and Bonnie Shulman. Their commitment to social justice has inspired my own.

—Neil Shulman

Medical literacy is the missing link in quality health care. Health education is just as important as the three R's, for without health, it's difficult to read, write, or do arithmetic.

—Neil Shulman

CONTENTS

TABLES AND FIGURES

ACKNOWLEDGMENTS

O UR HEARTFELT THANKS go the physicians, nurses, researchers and other professionals who personally shared their knowledge with us: Michael Kell, Thomas Hestor, Keith Woods, Sharni Sheehy, Hugh Moore, Gurinderjit Sidhu, Bruce Herschatter, John Ambri, Charles Gilbert, Charles Francis, Barry Silverman, William Mitch, Mark Stephen Travis, Joe Havlik, James Delcher, Mark Rosenberg, James Hunter, Stephanie Fox, Cathy Schnell, Lane Harrison, Debra Mlambo, Ira Bragg, Stacy Pelisero, Mary Stewart, David Grant, Joyce Dittmer, Ms. Thomas, Trish Grindell, Katheryn Tauber, Ira Schwartz, Kathy Berkowitz, Deb Sanden, Mae Clayton, Julie Feltham, Polly Clary, Melanie McLeod, Cam Langston, Lynn Humphrey, Patti Moore, Inginia Genao, Jada Bussby Jones, Murtaz Cassoubhoy, and Kena R. Norris.

Thanks also to these physicians and other health professionals who helped us to update the material for this new edition: Terry A. Jacobson W. Dallas Hall, Herbert R. Karp, Rita J. Louard,

Sam Newcom, Allan F. Platt, Jr., C. Magnus Nzerue, Sheldon Paul Kottle, Sureyya Hornston, Janet Cleveland, M. S., Janet Blair, and Alan Metzel .

We are grateful to Mark L. Walker for contributing our new chapter on violence.

We especially want to thank all the patients and families who educated us about their personal experiences, which helped us to develop the fictional case studies in this book. All names have been changed. We wish them many years of health and happiness. We also wish to thank those who gave us permission to use previously published figures to illustrate our text.

Although there are only three names on the cover of this book, the work could never have occurred without the diligent writing, editing, typing, indexing and proofreading talents of Robin Voss, Laurie E. Smith, Judith Repetti, Michelle Graye, Robert Fiske and Linda Rao. Thank you is not enough, but they are the only two words in the English language that come close to expressing our gratitude. In addition, thanks to Tam Lin Neville for her patient work in renewing permissions, and to Letitia Sweitzer and Lynn Aaron, both invaluable members of the team.

Furniss Holloway and Robert Fiske brought their exceptional talents to the final editing tasks.

Bert Stern has gone way beyond the call of duty in making this book happen. Bert is a good friend and a man of soul.

We also want to thank Pfizer Pharmaceuticals, Inc. for its gracious support of this book.

Putting this book together was no easy task. All the participants had other commitments, but were willing to sacrifice their time and talents and devote their energies to this worthwhile project.

PREFACE

BLACK MEN DIE at a younger age than any other race-sex group in America. All Americans should be concerned about this unfortunate public health fact. However, more important, African Americans have the right to know why black men suffer more and what can be done to improve their plight.

This newly updated version of the book is being published by Hilton Publishing Company, under the leadership of Hilton Hudson, an African American heart surgeon. I applaud Dr. Hudson and his committed staff. I hope every African American will join in their efforts by reading this book and sharing it with others. Knowledge provides the power, the power to overcome.

Neil Shulman, MD
Associate Professor, Emory University School of Medicine
Author of *Your Body's Red Light Warning Signals* and
Doc Hollywood

ONE

An Overview

This book's for you if you're a young man who thinks he can live forever without doing anything about it.

This book's for you if you're middle-aged and have begun to worry about your blood pressure.

This book's for you if you're a woman whose man isn't taking care of himself, and you fear that the two of you will lose all of your dreams if he gets ill.

This book's for you if you've begun to experience frequent chest pains and wonder what they mean but are afraid to find out.

This book's for you if you worry about the cancer you see all around you and wonder what you might do to keep it away from your own door.

This book's for you if you have several sex partners and have begun to worry about AIDS.

1

This book's for you if you fear the violence around you—or the violence inside you.

This book's for you if you love life and have dreams and know that you'll need to keep your good health in order to fulfill them.

BLACK MEN IN AMERICA live an average of 70 years, whereas white men live an average of 73 years. This means that, for all of our diversity as a people, and even though we live in every part of the country, the color of our skin determines that we black men are more likely to get ill and more likely to die of that illness than our friends in other racial groups.

Fortunately, good health isn't so much a matter of fate as it is a frame of mind. Too often, we think about our health only when we become ill. By that time, illness is costly—not only in money but also in lost time. To be sick can mean losing one's footing in the world for a while, and it can mean discomfort and pain as well. To be very sick is to submit to treatments that can themselves bring discomfort; it is to find oneself in a world of needles and tubes that have become necessary to our recovery and cure.

Men in general, and black men in particular, are inclined to avoid medical care unless they are seriously ill. We tend to tough it out, as if admitting to body weakness is to admit to weakness as a man. But, in fact, to be a strong African American man is to be responsible to those you love and to yourself. Taking care of yourself physically and mentally, we think, is an essential part of that responsibility.

Often, bad health is the result of bad choices. Not exercising, not eating right, ignoring those early warnings the body sends to

tell us that, unless we pay attention, there's going to be trouble—
these are all bad choices. Prevention is the best medicine, and
early diagnosis is a close second.

Remember, poor health can destroy not only your body but
also your dreams and goals. Many men who give all of their spirit
and heart to achieving their goals are unwilling to invest equally
in their bodies. But when they fall ill, their dreams can fall into
the dust.

KNOWLEDGE IS THE CURE

Your first step toward becoming an activist for your own good
health is to learn how your body works. Sure, sometimes what
your doctor has to tell you sounds like a foreign language. But
keep in mind that learning how your body works, as well as
what's going on when it doesn't work, is learning about yourself.
You're a wonder and a gift, body as well as soul. And once you
know a bit more about the mechanics of that gift, you'll be more
inclined to keep it running smoothly.

Have you ever wondered what your doctor sees when he
looks into your eyes? Or what she hears when she listens to your
heart and chest? Are you curious about why your blood vessels
can clog, or why normal cells can turn cancerous? Answers to
questions like these can lead you into a new appreciation of your
body. They can also teach you empowerment—empowerment to
take care of your own health.

In recent decades, African American men have become
empowered to make changes: The civil rights movement and the
Million Man March are but two examples. The time has come for
us to become empowered anew. Now the job is to learn about our

bodies as inseparable from our selves. Learning that, we can learn to keep our health, even to save our lives. In that way, we'll have taken a first step, a big step, toward eliminating the inequalities in the American health system. And in that way we'll be making the radical statement that we deserve to live as long as the other guys.

We don't pretend that the reasons behind the inequality in the health system are easy to discover or that they're all within our control. Some of them, we all know, stem from racism, and some are socioeconomic—poor access to medical care, poverty, bad environment, lack of awareness. Some are matters of diet— too much salt, fat, and cholesterol—and lifestyle.

Of course, this book can't change all that. It can only mark a beginning by making you aware of what your body needs in order to work as you want it to. And at least some of that aware- ness *is* easy: good diet, stress reduction, early detection and treat- ment of illness—that's the prescription needed to reverse the bad statistics. No, you can't become your own doctor. But you *can* do a lot to prevent yourself from getting ill, to know enough to get to a doctor when you need one, and to show to others what it means to live a healthy life.

HOW THIS BOOK CAN HELP

If you read this book from start to finish, you will learn all you need to know about health as well as about disease. Some of the benefits of that learning we've talked about already. But there are still others.

- You'll learn how to avoid poisonous substances that destroy the inner workings of the body.

- You'll learn how, by stretching and exercising your body, you can keep your cells healthy and your heart strong.

- You'll learn how to choose activities, friendships, and work environments that keep the mind calm and peaceful, and why that calm benefits the body.

- You'll learn how medicine can benefit you even if you come down with a serious disease—how dialysis can replace diseased kidneys; how heart specialists can open clogged blood vessels without surgery; how chemicals, radiation, and surgery can rid your body of cancerous cells.

- Finally, with the help of your new knowledge, if you *do* fall ill, you'll communicate more effectively with your doctor and medical team. In that way, you'll become the best kind of patient—one who understands the treatment options available to him. The patient who can make informed choices is the patient likely to get the best treatment and thus to have the best chance for recovery and cure.

A NEW HERO

Too often we look to heroes who *aren't* like ourselves—super athletes, super entertainment stars, the rich and the glamorous. Now it's time for a new hero—an ordinary man who takes care of his own body. He does so because he respects himself and believes that he *deserves* to be healthy. And he does so because he knows that by staying healthy he can love well and work well, and harvest his own dreams. You'll meet some of these new heroic black men in this book. Maybe, by the time you've finished reading, you'll find that you've become one of them.

TWO

Taking Control of Your Health

EACH OF US GETS only one life to live. In order to live that life to its fullest, we need to take care of our own health. The first step is to live a healthy lifestyle. It is important for us all to take good care of our bodies, not just when we're sick or recuperating, but also when *we're healthy.* The fact is, everything you put into your body and everything you do with your body has a direct impact on your health. By making simple lifestyle changes, people reap a multitude of health benefits, from lowering high blood pressure to helping to prevent cancer.

In this chapter, we talk about simple steps you can take to arm yourself against disease. When you eat right and exercise, you build your defenses against illness by equipping your body with the fuel it needs to heal itself and to prevent illness from taking its toll. Making changes is never easy, but when it comes to your good health, doing so could be a matter of life or death. So start with these simple guidelines for good health, and head down the path to a healthier, happier life.

7

EAT A HEALTHY DIET

The statistics tell the story: Black men are more susceptible to certain illnesses than white men. Why? One theory is that our diets are unhealthy. Traditional Southern food is often saltier and higher in fat than that of the North. Although blacks now live in all areas of the United States, many of our ancestors, at one time or another, lived in the South. So the traditional Southern diet still has an influence on the way we eat today.

Salt contributes to high blood pressure, a disorder that can lead to fatal consequences such as heart attacks, kidney failure, or stroke. Fat clogs our arteries and may also contribute to heart disease, stroke, and complications of diabetes and high blood pressure.

Often we get so busy that we seem to have no time to make a home-cooked meal for ourselves or our families. Instead, we stop at a fast-food restaurant on the way home from work or pick up a frozen TV dinner at the supermarket. Though these meals may be convenient, they also tend to be high in fat, calories, salt, sugar, and cholesterol.

Here's an idea: Instead of depending on foods already prepared for you, try following these simple guidelines to eating a healthy diet. You may find that eating right is easier and more delicious than you thought!

EAT FOODS LOW IN SATURATED FAT AND "BAD" CHOLESTEROL

Learn to read food labels for content. The most important information to look for is fat and cholesterol content.

As a rule of thumb, it's a good idea to reduce the amount of total fat you eat. There are three basic kinds of fats: saturated

FOODS TO CHOOSE WHEN YOU SHOP

Meat, poultry, fish, and shellfish

Lean cuts of meat
    Beef: eye of the round, top round
    Pork: tenderloin, sirloin, top loin
    Veal: shoulder, ground veal, cutlets, sirloin
    Lamb: leg-shank
Lean of extra lean ham and ground beef
Chicken or turkey (remove skin)
Fish
Shellfish

Dairy foods

Skim or 1 percent milk
Cheese* labeled "reduced fat," "low fat," "light," "part-skim," or
    "fat free"
Low fat or nonfat yogurt

Fats and oils

Margarine* (diet, tub, liquid)
Oils (like canola, corn, olive, peanut, safflower, or sesame oil)

Fruits and vegetables

Fruits: any fresh, frozen, canned, or dried
Vegetables: any fresh, frozen, or canned* without cream or
    cheese sauces
Fresh or frozen juices

continued on the next page

"Foods to Choose When You Shop," continued

Breads, cereals, pasta, rice and other grains, and dry peas and beans

Breads* (like whole wheat, rye, pumpernickel, or white)
Buns, dinner rolls, bagels, English muffins, pita breads*
Low fat crackers (like bread sticks or saltines)*
Tortillas
Hot and cold cereals* (except granola or muesli)
Pasta (like plain noodles, spaghetti, macaroni)
Rice
Dry peas and beans: black-eyed peas, chick peas, kidney beans,
     lentils, navy beans, soybeans, split peas
Refried beans made with vegetable oil instead of lard

Sweets and snacks

Low fat cookies: animal crackers, devil's food cookies, fig and other
     fruit bars, ginger snaps, graham crackers, vanilla or lemon
     wafers
Angel food and other low fat cakes
Frozen yogurt, fruit ices, ice milk, sherbet
Pudding (make it with skim or 1 percent milk), gelatin desserts
Popcorn without butter, pretzels, baked tortilla chips*

* If you are watching your sodium intake, be sure to check the label to find low-
  sodium types.

Reprinted from "Step-by Step: Eating to Lower Your High Cholesterol," National
Institute of Health, National Heart, Lung, and Blood Institute, 1994.

(bad), polyunsaturated (better), and monounsaturated (good). Saturated fats clog your arteries and are unhealthy. If you *have* to eat fat, monounsaturated fats are much better for your body.

Check food labels to find out what kind of fat and cholesterol they contain. Many people know their cholesterol level number (the target is under 200), but few people actually know what this number means. Truth is, cholesterol, the waxy, yellowish material found in your body's organs, plays a valuable role in your body. It is the foundation for all cells in the body; it aids in digestion and produces hormones. However, as you probably know, cholesterol also can cause atherosclerosis (cholesterol buildup on the walls of your arteries), which can lead to cardiovascular disease.

On the surface of your heart rest three blood vessels the size of straws. If something as small as a pea gets in one of these straws, it can close off the artery and cause a heart attack. "Bad" cholesterol (see below) can do just that, by breaking off from the surface of your arteries and getting into your bloodstream, so as to block your smaller blood vessels entirely. This is why many studies show that the higher your cholesterol level, the greater your risk of coronary heart disease and stroke.

Cholesterol is divided into two major groups: high-density lipoprotein (HDL) and low-density lipoprotein (LDL). HDL is considered "good" cholesterol because it helps eliminate bad cholesterol from the circulatory system. The higher your HDL, the lower your risk of a heart attack. (Exercise or weight loss, by the way, may raise your HDL levels.) Smoking, on the other hand, lowers your HDL level.

LDL cholesterol, conversely, can be dangerous. The higher your LDL level, the greater your risk of heart disease.

CLASSIFCATION
TOTAL AND HDL-CHOLESTEROL[*]

Total Cholesterol

Desirable Blood Cholesterol	Borderline-High Blood Cholesterol	High Blood Cholesterol
less than 200 mg/dL	200–239 mg/dL	240 mg/dL and above

HDL-Cholesterol

		Low HDL-Cholesterol
		Less than 35 mg/dL

* These levels are for anyone 20 years of age or older

CLASSIFCATION
LDL-CHOLESTEROL[*]

Desirable	Borderline-High Risk	High Risk
less than 130 mg/dL	130–159 mg/dL	160 mg/dL and above

* These levels are for anyone 20 years of age or older without heart disease. A person with heart disease should have an LDL level of 100 mg/dL or less.

Reprinted from "Step-by Step: Eating to Lower Your High Cholesterol," National Institute of Health, National Heart, Lung, and Blood Institute, 1994.

HOW CHOLESTEROL FORMS ON THE WALL OF AN ARTERY

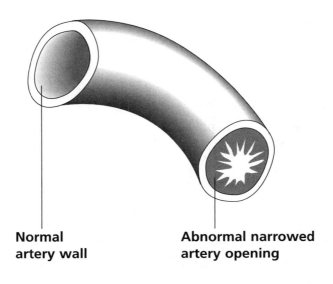

Normal artery wall   **Abnormal narrowed artery opening**

Reprinted from "Coronary Artery Disease Explained," NHLBI

Maintaining a high ratio of good HDL to bad LDL is more important than lowering your overall cholesterol level. A 10-year study conducted by the National Institutes of Health looked at 3,806 men between the ages of 35 and 59 with cholesterol levels above 265 mg/dl. This study confirmed that dietary cholesterol is largely responsible for atherosclerosis and that reducing cholesterol will definitely lower heart disease risk. (We will discuss this type of heart disease further in Chapter 4.) "If we can get everyone to lower their cholesterol by 10 to 15 percent by cutting down on fat and cholesterol in their diet, heart attack deaths in this country will decrease by 30 percent," concluded Dr. Robert Levy, the cardiologist who helped coordinate the 10-year study.

When it comes to fat and cholesterol, here are some additional tips to remember:

- *Avoid eating butter, margarine, and oils high in cholesterol and saturated fat.* Instead, choose a margarine with a liquid vegetable oil as the first ingredient. Tip: A tub of margarine contains more polyunsaturated fat than a stick of margarine. Take advantage of the "light" margarines that are now available. Spend a couple of extra cents and save your body the cost of clogged arteries.

- *Use liquid vegetable oils whenever possible.* In recipes calling for one cup of solid shortening, substitute 3/4 cup of liquid vegetable oil; replace 1/2 cup shortening with 1/3 cup vegetable oil. When cooking foods on the stove or in a wok, use canola or olive oil, both of which are high in monounsaturated (good) fat. Remember to use all oils sparingly since they're high in calories!

- *Use low-fat or nonfat dairy products.* Although dairy products have been touted as healthy because they contain calcium, they also can have a high fat content. So choose low-fat options, such as skim milk and nonfat yogurt, whenever possible. Choose cheeses that have less than 5 grams of fat. (High-fat cheeses can add inches to your waistline and also clog your arteries.) On the other hand, fat-free foods such as broccoli and leafy green vegetables can provide you with all the calcium your body needs.

- *When cooking, substitute low-fat or nonfat dairy products for high-fat recipe ingredients.* For example, you can use low-fat or nonfat yogurt for cream and mayonnaise.

- *Avoid eating egg yolks.* If you like eggs, check your supermarket for egg substitutes, which are a healthier alternative because they contain egg whites with coloring rather than egg yolks. (The yellow yolk in eggs is high in cholesterol, whereas egg whites are high in protein and low in cholesterol.) You can use egg substitutes for baking or to make scrambled eggs or omelets.

- *Enjoy a fruit cup.* Another healthy alternative to eggs for breakfast is fresh fruit. A fruit salad made with strawberries, grapes, bananas, melons, and oranges can be a delicious and energizing way to start your day. If you can't give up eggs, limit your intake to no more than three per week. And choose egg whites over egg yolks.

EAT FRESH VEGETABLES

Although we may hate to admit it, our mothers were right when they told us to eat our vegetables! As with fruit, vegetables require little to no preparation. All you have to do is rinse, peel, or cut to your liking and munch away! Most types of veggies are delicious raw. Since they make such a great snack on the go, it's easy to take a few carrots or celery sticks to work with you. There are so many different kinds of vegetables: If you think you hate vegetables, go to the supermarket and buy something you've never eaten before. You'll be pleasantly surprised.

Fresh vegetables are also delicious in a salad. If you prefer cooked vegetables, steam them lightly over a pan of water or in the microwave. Make sure to cover them to trap the steam and nutrients. Be careful not to overcook them though because vegetables retain most of their flavor and nutrients only when they

MAKING RECIPES HEALTHIER

Most recipes can be modified to reduce the amount of sugar, salt and/or fat called for in the ingredient list.

Here are some tips:

To Reduce Salt

Choosing Snack Foods
Look for crackers, chips, popcorn, and pretzels that are unsalted or low in salt and that have 1 or 2 grams of fat per serving.

Cutting Salt When Preparing Foods
- Use low-sodium or reduced-sodium soy sauce, steak sauce, catsup, and barbecue sauce.
- Dilute regular soy sauce with an equal amount of water or wine.
- Cook with unsalted butter or margarine, or use vegetable oil, which is salt-free.
- Substitute chicken or turkey for prosciutto, ham, or other salty, cured meats.
- Cook with reduced-sodium cheese, salad dressing, and mayonnaise.
- Use lemon juice, flavored vinegars, pepper, garlic, and other herbs and spices in place of salt.
- Use garlic, onion, and celery powders in place of garlic, onion, and celery salts.
- Skip the salt when preparing pasta, rice, vegetables, and hot cereal.
- Omit salt in recipes. In some recipes, you can use half the amount of salt called for. In other recipes, you can leave the salt out altogether. Be careful, though,—many baking recipes, such as those made with yeast, need salt for the recipe to work.

To Reduce Sugar

- You can reduce the sugars called for in many baking recipes by 1/4 to 1/2 without affecting the quality. A general guideline is to use 1/4 cup or less of added sugars for each cup of flour.
- Fresh fruit is a natural replacement for all or part of the sugar in a recipe. Try applesauce in baked goods, fresh fruit instead of syrup on pancakes, and fruit juice in salad dressings. Be aware that fruit juice or fruit juice concentrates have more nutrients than sugar, such as vitamin C, but they provide the same amount of calories and carbohydrate, and they raise blood glucose about as high as sugar does.

Reprinted with permission from American Diabetes Association, *How to Cook for People with Diabetes* (1996).

SOURCES OF SATURATED FAT AND CHOLESTEROL

Animal fat	Egg and egg-yolk solids	Palm kernel oil
Bacon fat	Ham fat	Palm oil
Beef fat	Hardened fat or oil	Pork fat
Butter	Hydrogenated vegetable oil	Vegetable oil (avoid
Cheese	Turkey fat	coconut or palm oils)
Chicken fat	Lamb fat	Cocoa butter
Coconut	Lard	Vegetable shortening
Coconut oil	Meat fat	Whole-milk solids
Cream		

Reprinted from National Institute of Health, National Heart, Lung and Blood Institute: "Step by Step: Eating to Lower Your High Blood Cholesterol," February 1999 are cooked lightly. Avoid boiling or cooking vegetables with fat. Did you know that boiling and overcooking actually remove the good nutrients your body needs? And cooking with butter or oil can ruin the natural goodness of vegetables!

When fresh vegetables aren't available, use frozen; the nutrient content comes closest to fresh. Canned vegetables may contain preservatives and tend to be high in sodium although they can also be more affordable. If you prefer to buy canned vegetables, choose those that are labeled *low in sodium.*

EAT MORE FRESH FRUIT

Most people like fruit. It's sweet, easy to eat, and convenient. Best of all, fruit is one of the most healthy things you could ever eat! By eating a variety of fruits and vegetables, you can get many of the vitamins your body needs. Since there's no preparation involved, you can pick up a piece of fruit between appointments, on the way to work or as an evening snack.

Fruit is filled with natural carbohydrates and fiber, which your body desperately needs to function properly and supply you with energy. Try to eat at least five servings of fruits and vegetables every day.

EAT WHOLE GRAINS

Whole grain breads and pastas, rice, beans, and grains are the foundation of a good diet. When eating carbohydrates, such as pasta or bread, choose whole grain alternatives. Always look for whole wheat products because they have more fiber and nutrients. When a product is labeled "wheat," it isn't necessarily made from whole wheat grains. If you're in doubt, check the label. If caramel coloring has been added, there's a good chance the actual wheat content in the product is low.

Whole wheat bread and pastas teem with nutrients and fiber. *Oat bran* products (including oatmeal) help decrease the bad cholesterol in your blood system, which helps to prevent cancer and heart disease. The fiber in wheat bran also helps to prevent cancer by helping your body process the food you eat. White bread, on the other hand, is almost devoid of fiber and natural nutrients. Try to eat natural grain products several times each day.

REDUCE SALT

In American culture, salt has become something of a flavor saver. If something tastes bad or bland, we just shake some salt on it. But we aren't born liking the taste of salty foods. In fact, we acquire all of our food tastes and cravings. If you never introduce salt into a newborn baby's diet, for example, you reduce the chances that the child will crave salt as an adult.

It wasn't until fairly recently—the 1950s—that we discovered the harmful effects of eating too much salt. Because it may contribute to high blood pressure, we should try to limit our sodium intake. (See Chapter 3 for a more thorough discussion of high blood pressure in black men.) Unfortunately, junk food and snack food such as peanuts, pretzels, and potato chips contain a great deal of salt.

The first step you need to take to avoid salt is to remove the saltshaker from the kitchen or dining room table. Then stock up on tasty and healthy spices that you can use as substitutes. Try pepper, basil, oregano, garlic, Cajun spices or spice preparations, such as Mrs. Dash.

HIGH-SALT FOODS

Bacon

Baking powder

Baking soda

Beans (canned)

Bouillon (beef or chicken)

Bologna

Buttermilk (commercial)

Canned meats (beef stew, chili)

Canned soups

Canned vegetables

Cheese

Chitlins (pickled)

Fast foods

Frozen prepared foods

Hamburger

Ham hock

Hog maw (pickled)

Hot dogs

Instant grits

Instant oatmeal

Ketchup

Luncheon meats

Monosodium glutamate (MSG)

Mustard

Olives

Pickles (dill or onion)

Pig's feet (pickled)

Pizza

Pot pies

Potato chips

Pretzels

Salted nuts

Saltines

Sauerkraut

Sausage

Seasonings*

Self-rising flour or meal

Soda crackers

Soy sauce

Steak sauces

Tomato juice

TV dinners

* Garlic salt, seasoning salt, onion salt, allspice, MSG, teriyaki, lemon pepper, pre-mixed seasonings for meat, poultry, and fish

COOKING WITH HERBS AND SPICES

Herbs and spices can flavor your food in place of salt, fat, or sugar. One way to make herbs and spices release their flavor is to heat them. You can do this by sautéing them; boiling them in soups, stews, or sauces; or putting them on meats or vegetables before cooking. When adding herbs and spices to soups or stews, do so during the last hour of cooking to preserve their flavor.

Another way to release the flavor of herbs and spices is to crush them before you use them. You can crush herbs and spices with a mortar and pestle, blender, or chopper.

Soaking herbs and spices in a cold liquid also releases their flavor. But this takes much longer—days and weeks. This method can be used to make flavored oils and vinegars, salad dressings, and marinades.

If a recipe calls for fresh herbs and you will be using dried herbs, use 1/3 the amount called for. If a recipe calls for dried herbs and you will be using fresh herbs, use three times the amount called for. If you are trying an herb or spice for the first time, start by adding 1/4 teaspoon of dried herbs or 1 teaspoon of chopped fresh herbs for every four servings of food.

Buy fresh herbs no more than a few days before you plan to use them. Keep them wrapped in a damp paper towel in a plastic bag. Buy dried herbs and spices in small amounts, because they lose flavor the longer they sit around.

Reprinted with permission from American Diabetes Association, "How to Cook for People with Diabetes" (1996), pp. 21-22.

REDUCE YOUR INTAKE OF FRIED FOOD

If you do go to fast-food restaurants, try to order food that has not been fried. For example, many restaurants now offer broiled or baked chicken sandwiches or salads as part of their menu. When you're cooking at home, use the same rule: Avoid eating fried food. Not only does frying require soaking the food in grease, but the cooking process locks the fat inside. So when you eat fried food, the fat is more likely to clog your arteries, add inches to your waistline, and put you at higher risk of heart disease. Before biting into food cooked in oil, think of all that grease going straight to your heart, then decide if you really want to do that to your body.

LIMIT INTAKE OF RED MEAT

Red meat, such as hamburgers and steaks, is filled with saturated fat and is high in bad cholesterol. Unfortunately, many of us have come to enjoy red meat as a regular part of our diet. Contrary to what was once taught, meat and potatoes do not make a healthy dinner after all. Many of us were told as children that red meat makes our bodies and muscles strong. After all, meat contains iron and protein, right?

Surprisingly, your body doesn't need as much protein as we once thought. Excess protein can actually decrease the absorption of other important nutrients in your body. Besides, you can get plenty of protein from healthy, delicious foods such as beans, fish, chicken (with the skin removed and not fried), and low-fat dairy products.

When you eat fatty red meat (such as fatty hamburgers and prime rib), you may be substantially shortening your life, especially since that food has been closely linked to heart disease, the leading killer of black Americans. If you can, give up red meat altogether. If you can't give it up, make a committed effort to eating meat only once in a while. Be sure to limit portion sizes to only 3 to 5 ounces.

EAT FISH INSTEAD OF RED MEAT

If you're looking for a healthy substitute for red meat, try fish. Fish is significantly lower in fat than red meat. Ask your medical professional for more information about the healthy benefits of eating fish. Be careful, though, to limit the amount of shellfish you eat (such as shrimp or lobster) since these tend to contain a lot of cholesterol.

There are many delicious kinds of fish, so take some time to experiment to find those that appeal to you most. If you're looking for a good substitute for red meat, swordfish and tuna steaks offer a dense texture, similar to red meat. And they taste delicious! Ask the attendant at your local fish market or the fish counter in your supermarket for ways to cook these and other fish. Just don't fry them or cook them with butter and oils, or coat them with fat, such as mayonnaise, butter, and tartar sauce!

NO MORE JUNK FOOD

The junk food industry makes a great deal of money by making unhealthy foods seem very attractive, so before you buy pre-processed foods, do your research. Pretzels and crackers with less than 2 grams of fat per serving are excellent choices for snack foods. Always check the sodium and fat content of other foods you buy as well. Most junk foods contain large amounts of salt, sugar, and fat. A good rule is if it doesn't grow, don't eat it. If that rule doesn't work, at least think about how a certain food may be benefiting your body. Soda pop, though never proved to cause cancer, offers your body absolutely nothing of value. If it's not helping, it may be part of the problem.

Fast food is one of the biggest contributors to the health problems facing our black community, especially in the South, where fast food mirrors the typical high-fat, high-salt Southerner's diet. Fast food is appealing everywhere because it's quick, readily available, and affordable. Many people today have less time to prepare food for themselves and their families, and as a result, we're all getting less good nutrition. But there's a price to pay for that speed and convenience.

When you purchase fast food, you're getting a lot more for your money than you realize. In addition to hamburgers and French fries, you're getting huge doses of cholesterol, fat, sodium, and calories. American adults should consume no more than 30 percent of their total calories from fat (67 grams on a 2,000 calorie diet) and no more than 2,400 milligrams of sodium (about 1 1/4 teaspoons) per day, according to the American Heart Association's dietary guidelines. If you go to Burger King and eat a Double Whopper with Cheese, you've eaten 67 grams of fat and 1,460 grams of sodium—more than half the limit. Throw in a king-size order of French fries and you've surpassed your daily fat and sodium limit in only one meal!

Let's say you like chicken more than hamburgers, so you order a chicken sandwich with mayo and king-size onion rings. Maybe you think you've made the "healthy" choice because you've chosen chicken rather than red meat. Instead, you've just consumed 73 grams of fat in one meal alone—more than your days' limit. You've also consumed 1,310 calories and 2,280 milligrams of sodium (just under your allotment for the day). After that one fast-food meal, the only way you can keep within healthy dietary limits is not to eat for the next couple of days. (We can all imagine how unhealthy, not to mention difficult, fasting can be!) As we blacks rely more and more on fast food for our meals it's no wonder that obesity is a growing problem in the African American community.

The fact that fast-food restaurants are so popular and prevalent doesn't mean that fast food is good for you. Fast-food businesses—like everyone else—are out to make money. If you buy their unhealthy food, they'll keep selling it. Many fast-food chains insist that their food is indeed healthy and getting healthier. It's true that some of them now offer lower fat options and salads. Overall, however, most of the food served by these restaurants is extremely unhealthy.

Here's a tip: Before eating or drinking something, always ask yourself, "How is this helping my body?" If no answer comes to mind, ask yourself, "Is there something else I can eat or drink instead that will give my body what it really needs?" If there is, it might be worth your while to go out of your way and make the healthy choice. A little extra effort now can save you a lot of suffering later. It's difficult to change lifelong eating habits. But if you care enough about your health, you'll find the motivation you need to modify your diet.

DRINK LOTS OF WATER AND FRESH FRUIT JUICE

Our bodies are comprised of more than 60 percent water. That's a lot! To maintain good health, we need to help our bodies maintain that proportion. You may be dehydrated more often than

FAT, CHOLESTEROL, CALORIES, AND SODIUM CONTENT IN JUNK FOODS

Snack (1 ounce	Saturated Fat (grams)	Cholesterol (mgs)	Total Fat (grams)	Calories from Fat (%)	Total Calories	Sodium (mgs)
Pretzels, salted (1 oz. is about 5 twists, 3 1/4 x 2 1/4 x 1/4 in.)	0.2	0	1.0	8	108	486
Popcorn, air popped without salt (1 oz. is about 3 1/2 cups)	0.2	0	1.2	10	108	1
Tortilla chips, lower fat (light) nacho flavor	0.8	1	4.3	31	126	284
Corn Chips	1.3	0	9.5	56	153	179
Popcorn, popped with oil and salt (1 oz. is about 2 1/2 cups)	1.4	0	8.0	51	142	251
Tortilla chips, nacho flavor	1.4	1	7.3	47	141	201
Trail mix (1 oz. is about 1/5 cups	1.6	0	8.3	57	131	65
Potato chips	3.1	0	9.8	58	152	168

Reprinted from NIHLBI, "Step by Step: Eating to Lower Your Blood Cholesterol" (February 1999), p. 10.

CHOOSE A HEALTHIER SNACK

Snack on...

Air-popped popcorn with no butter, unsalted pretzels

Hard candy, jelly beans

Bagels, raisin toast, or English muffins with margarine or jelly

Low-fat cookies (such as fig bars, vanilla wafers, ginger snaps)

Fruits, vegetables

Fruit juices and drinks

Frozen yogurt, sherbet, ice pops

Instead of...

Popcorn with butter

Chocolate bars

Doughnuts, Danish pastry

Cake, cookies, brownies

Milk shakes, eggnogs, floats

Ice cream

Reprinted from National Institute of Health: *Eat Right to Lower Your High Blood Cholesterol,* March 1992.

you realize. Without an adequate amount of water in our cells, our bodies have a tough time functioning. It's like expecting a car to keep on moving when it's almost out of gas!

The way to help our bodies maintain 60 percent of water is simple: Drink water! Some experts say we should drink between 8 and 10 glasses of water each day. If you live in an area where your tap water is contaminated, you might want to drink bottled water or use a water filter. Some authorities say that we can get away with drinking less water if we eat a lot of foods with a high water content, such as fruits and vegetables. Remember, however, that cooking removes the naturally high levels of water from these foods.

Drinking fresh fruit juice also boosts your body's water content. If you have a choice between eating an orange and drinking orange juice, it's usually healthier to choose the orange because it contains fiber. If you're looking for something healthy to drink, though, 100 percent fruit juice is a great alternative to soda or fruit drinks. (Read labels carefully. Although fruit drinks may claim to contain real fruit juice, they often contain high levels of sugar and corn syrup, which decrease the fruit and vitamins you're receiving and increase your intake of sugar and empty calories.)

Not all drinks boost your water content. Those that contain caffeine or alcohol can actually dehydrate water from your cells, reducing your body's water content. To be safe, make a habit of drinking lots of water.

A WORD ON DIETS

Overweight people tend to have more heart problems than other folks because they generally don't get enough exercise—an important factor for a healthy heart and body. If you're carrying around extra weight, you're making your heart work harder. If you're already sedentary, you should not put additional strain on your body with unnecessary weight.

Nevertheless, don't get lured into going on one of the quickie, cure-all fad diets that are so popular today. By going on and off diets, you not only put your body in a dangerous habit of gaining and losing weight, but you may also lose muscle and actually weaken your immune system and your ability to burn fat. Better to change your eating habits and commit to a lifetime of healthy eating. You'll lose weight gradually, naturally, and healthfully.

Try to follow the guidelines in this chapter every single day, for the rest of your life. Most important, limit your fat intake and

OVERWEIGHT TRENDS BY SEX AND RACE*

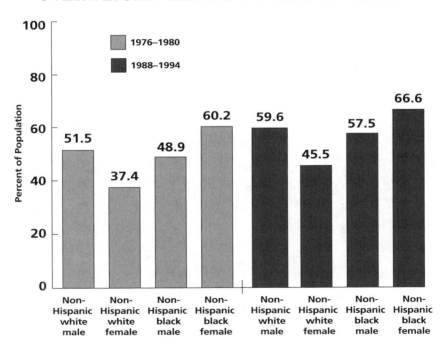

* The Center for Disease Control defines "overweight" as greater than or equal to 25kgs/m². Their samples drew from people in the 20-74 year old age range.

Chart based on Flegal, K.M., et al., "Overweight and Obesity in the United States: Prevalence and Trends, 1960-94," *Int. J. Obes. Relat. Metab. Disord.* XXII (1998), 39-47.

eat lots of natural grain products, fresh fruits, and vegetables. Remember, most fruits and vegetables contain no fat and actually equip your body with the fuel it needs to burn fat more efficiently. The best thing about fruits and vegetables is that you can eat a lot without risking gaining weight.

Also remember not to cover healthy foods with high-fat dressings or cheese, or with fat and cholesterol by frying them. Fried vegetables, such as French fries, can be particularly misleading. You may think you're doing something good for your body because you're eating vegetables, but because these foods are fried, you're actually doing more harm than good. Try using lemon juice, herbs, and spices for seasonings. If you have to use a dressing, make sure it's low in fat or, better yet, fat-free. It may be a good idea to work with a physician, nurse, dietitian or health educator to design the most healthy diet for you. Your doctor can also help you to develop a personalized exercise program that meets your needs. Don't, however, be suckered into spending lots of money on quick cures. By following the guidelines outlined in this chapter, you are more likely to have a healthy body for life, not just a few months of thinness. In addition to healthy food, exercise is very important when it comes to losing weight and maintaining good health; we should all make exercise a regular part of our lives. Later in this chapter, we'll discuss how to begin.

STOP SMOKING

Smoking is another bad habit some of us use to reduce stress. Although smoking may seem like a quick fix, its long-term consequences can be deadly. *Smoking is the single most preventable cause of premature death*: It causes lung cancer and contributes to heart disease and stroke—the three leading killers of black men. If all black men were to stop using tobacco, we could avoid thousands of deaths every year. If you smoke, stop. If you don't smoke, good for you! Never start.

The U.S. Surgeon General has called nicotine an addictive drug for three reasons. First, when used in small amounts, nicotine produces pleasurable feelings that make you want to smoke more. Second, when people try to quit smoking, they suffer both physical and psychological withdrawal symptoms—such as nervousness, headaches, and sleeplessness. Third, nicotine affects brain and central nervous system chemistry, which explains how the habit affects a person's mood and feelings. The addictive nature of smoking makes it so difficult for many of us to quit.

If you're trying to quit, you may have heard about alternative methods such as cigarettes with less tar and nicotine, as well as chewing tobacco and snuff. Unfortunately, these are *not* safe alternatives. Because smokeless tobacco contains nicotine (the same drug found in cigarettes), it's harmful, too. In fact, snuff dippers take in over 10 times more cancer-causing substances (called nitrosamines) than cigarette smokers. These substances are absorbed through the lining of the mouth and can cause sores and white patches that often lead to oral cancers.

Studies show that menthol cigarettes may be even more dangerous to your health and that blacks tend to smoke more of these cigarettes than whites. Menthol smokers can inhale more deeply or hold the smoke inside longer than smokers of nonmenthol cigarettes. This may be a reason why blacks, who actually smoke fewer cigarettes a day, are more likely than whites to die from smoking-related diseases such as lung cancer, heart disease, and stroke.

RISKS OF SMOKING

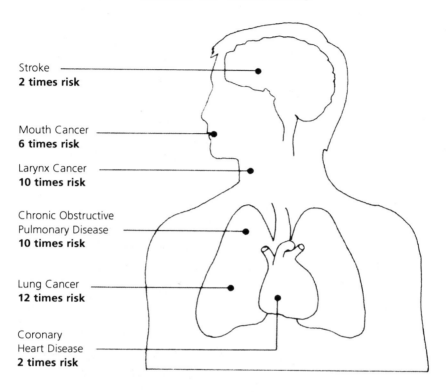

Stroke
2 times risk

Mouth Cancer
6 times risk

Larynx Cancer
10 times risk

Chronic Obstructive
Pulmonary Disease
10 times risk

Lung Cancer
12 times risk

Coronary
Heart Disease
2 times risk

Reprinted from National Institute of Health, National Heart, Lung, and Blood Institute, "Nurses: Help Your Patients Stop Smoking," January 1993.

In addition to its many other drawbacks, cigarette smoking can also be harmful to your arteries. If there's one thing that nearly all doctors agree on, it's that smoking remains the most important controllable risk factor for cardiovascular disease. If you smoke, you have a 70 percent greater coronary heart disease death and stroke rate, and a two- to four-times greater risk of coronary heart disease and sudden death (from abrupt loss of

CONTROL YOUR WITHDRAWAL SYMPTOMS

Withdrawal Symptom	Things You Might Do Instead
Craving for cigarettes	Do something else; take slow, deep breaths; tell yourself, "Don't do it."
Anxiety	Take slow, deep breaths; don't drink caffeine drinks; do other things.
Irritability	Walk; take slow, deep breaths; do other things.
Trouble sleeping	Don't drink caffeine drinks in the evening; don't take naps during the day; imagine something relaxing like a favorite spot.
Lack of concentration	Do something else; take a walk.
Tiredness	Exercise; get plenty of rest.
Dizziness	Sit or lie down when needed; know that it will pass.
Headaches	Relax; take mild pain medication as needed.
Coughing	Sip water.
Constipation	Drink lots of water; eat high-fiber foods such as vegetables and fruits.
Hunger	Eat well-balanced meals; eat low-calorie snacks; drink cold water.

Reprinted from National Institute of Health, National Heart, Lung, and Blood Institute, "Nurses: Help Your Patients Stop Smoking," January 1993.

heart function) than nonsmokers. Studies show that your risk of death from heart disease will greatly decrease after you quit smoking; in fact, some studies have shown a benefit within two years after quitting, whereas others have suggested that your risk of death will gradually decrease over several years.

Smoking doesn't affect just the smoker; it affects everyone around him—including nonsmokers. Studies show that the pas-

HOW MANY CALORIES ARE YOU BURNING?

Activity	Total Calories used per Hour*
Ballroom dancing	125–310
Walking slowly (2.5 mph)	210–230
Brisk walking (4 mph)	250–345
Jogging (6 mph)	315–480
Cycling (9 mph)	315–480
Tennis	315–480
Basketball	480–625
Swimming	480–625
Cross-country skiing	480–625

*Expenditure in calories by a 150-pound person.

Reprinted with permission of the Georgia Egg Commission: *Your Wellness Guide to a Healthy Lifestyle*.

sive smoke contains the same chemicals as the smoke inhaled by smokers and actually gives off larger amounts of cancer-causing substances.

Ask your doctor about available resources to help you quit. Many options are available, including support groups, medications, and nicotine patches and gums. Although quitting can be very difficult, chances are that once you experience what it is like to have smoke-free lungs, you'll agree it was worth the struggle.

STOP SUBSTANCE ABUSE

Smoking is not the only escape we use when we're stressed out. Some of us enjoy cocktails, beer, or drugs such as cocaine or marijuana. Although these substances may make you feel good, the effect they have on your body is devastating; in fact, these "feel good" potions may be slowly killing you. Drink after drink, drag after drag, your cells are dying, one by one, leading to disease and heartache for you and your loved ones.

Drinking alcohol, though legal for adults, is one of the most dangerous habits we can develop. A drink every now and then may not hurt, but alcohol is addictive and it's easy to become hooked. A leading killer of black men is cirrhosis of the liver, which is caused by heavy drinking. Because substance abuse is such a serious health problem, we have dedicated an entire chapter to this issue.

If substance abuse is of concern to you, read Chapter 10 carefully. Then, confide in your doctor. Together, you can fight your habit—whatever it may be. By working with a medical professional and making up your mind to change, you will find that good health can be yours again.

EXERCISE EVERY DAY

You don't have to look far for signs that exercise is good for you. In fact, all you have to do is turn on the TV. You'll be confronted with television shows and ads all touting the benefits of a physically active lifestyle. No matter how commercial these ploys may be, the message they're sending is a valid one: Exercise is good for you. Exercise reduces your risk of heart disease by decreasing the amount of LDL (bad) cholesterol in your cardiovascular system, while it increases your HDL (good) cholesterol. Working out also helps you maintain or lose weight, increases the strength of your heart muscle, increases the amount of enzymes in your body that burn fat, helps reduce stress, improves circulation, decreases elevated blood pressure, decreases your percentage of body fat, and increases the amount of muscle mass in your body.

Aerobic exercise, such as walking, jogging, biking, or swimming, uses a lot of energy and strengthens your heart and lungs. Regular aerobic exercise also improves circulation throughout your body and improves your body's ability to use oxygen. Exercise also builds energy levels, reduces stress and tension, helping you to relax and sleep better.

It's never too late to start an exercise program; just check with your doctor before you begin. Most physicians will gladly assist you in planning your personal fitness program. (Their advice is important because some exercises, such as weightlifting, can be quite strenuous and aren't a good option for everyone, especially those people with high blood pressure or coronary heart disease.) Regardless of the exercise program you choose, make sure it's something you enjoy because, above all else, exercise should be fun.

According to the American Heart Association, any exercise you undertake should begin with a warm-up period, which prepares your body for the exercise to follow. The next phase of exercise, which is more vigorous, will make your heart stronger and bring more oxygen into your body, both of which will make you feel better.

Exercise at least five times a week for a minimum of 30 minutes a day—and remember that physical activity doesn't necessarily need to be vigorous to confer cardiovascular benefits. For example, moderate activity, such as brisk walking, can be just as beneficial. Just remember to cool down slowly and completely after you exercise.

And don't overdo it! Take it slow, and be patient with your body. As time passes, you'll be able to do more; just let this process happen naturally. Everyone's body is different. Listen to yours to learn when and when not to push yourself harder. Remember: Exercise should be fun because, just like a healthy diet, it's a habit that should last for the rest of your life. Think of exercise as time to play and enjoy it!

REDUCE YOUR STRESS

*The American Heritage Dictionary of the English Lan*guage describes stress as "a mentally or emotionally disruptive or upsetting condition occurring in response to adverse external influences and capable of affecting physical health, usually characterized by increased heart rate, a rise in blood pressure, muscular tension, irritability and depression." In other words, stress, when out of control, can cause a great deal of emotional and physical damage. Learning to cope with these pressures is a key factor in maintaining a healthy lifestyle.

Whereas exercise makes your immune system stronger, excess stress can make you more vulnerable to disease. Once you're sick, stress can also weaken your body's ability to fight back. Blacks, in particular, suffer from a great deal of stress that often begins at childhood. Some experts think the excess stress is due to the racial discrimination we experience in our social and work surroundings. Think, for example, how you feel when several white people cross the street when they see you walking toward them at night. Aren't you frustrated when a police officer stops your car to check your driver's license for no apparent reason? Or when you can't get a taxi to stop and pick you up? You're a black man. Our skin color often puts us at a disadvantage. Depending on where we live, events such as these may happen quite often, and when they do, they can cause a lot of stress.

The real question is: Are you able to rise above these injustices? Do you feel victimized and angry when you're mistreated because of the color of your skin? Or do you accept these insults as a challenge to prove your worth and integrity? Carefully watch the way your body reacts when you're in stressful situations because your overall health and well-being are intricately tied to your state of mind. Becoming aware of anger and distress can be the first step toward controlling it. And you don't have to do all the work alone. You have many resources for coping with the strains of daily living; seek the objective advice from a friend, counselor, minister, psychologist, or psychiatrist.

Black men are very vulnerable to stress since, even though resources may be available, they may not have learned how to seek social support to deal with challenging situations. For starters, it's a good idea to develop emotionally intimate relationships with at least two or three people—men or women with whom you can share your deepest secrets and on whom you can count for support.

You can also release excess stress by exercising regularly and by taking advantage of the many entertainment options available. Get involved in any activity that brings you pleasure: Take a walk, get involved in a game, call a friend, do anything to remove yourself from a stressful situation and relax and enjoy yourself. The situation may still be there when you come back, but the break will help you deal with it better.

Take constructive action to make your life more relaxed. If your job seems to be a constant source of stress, try incorporating the aforementioned stress-reducing strategies into your daily life. Start a hobby or sport that you can look forward to doing at the end of a long working day. If you find yourself getting upset at work, make a conscious effort to think about things that make you happy outside of work. Use your coffee and bathroom breaks to go for a brisk walk outside.

If you've tried all these techniques and none of them seems to be working, consider what options you have. If it's your job that causes you constant stress, maybe it's time to consider changing jobs. If constant caretaking of children or an elderly person is stressful, ask a friend or family member to take over for a week.

Whatever you do, don't attempt to relieve your stress by drinking, smoking, overeating, or using drugs. Although such indulgences may soothe your tension for a while, in the long run, they'll make it worse by harming your health and further complicating your life.

Only you can take control of your own level of stress, and to accomplish this task, you need to pay attention to the signals you're getting from your mind and body. If you're under too much stress, there are many techniques you can use, such as diaphragmatic breathing, meditation (incorporating any spiritual beliefs you have), and guided imagery. Worrying too much over day-to-day problems can jeopardize your health, so when you feel stressed out, do something about it. For more information on stress reduction techniques, read *Beyond the Relaxation Response*, by Herbert Benson, M.D. (Berkley Publishing Group, 1994), or *The Healthy Mind Healthy Body Workbook*, by David S. Sobel, M.D., and Robert Ornstein, Ph.D. (I S H K Book Service, May 1997).

GET SUPPORT

Most important, get your family and loved ones involved. If you're making changes in your lifestyle, it's important that those people close to you understand and support the changes you are making. Turning to them can turn a difficult, solitary task into a loving and joyful one. If your wife, mother, or partner does most of the cooking in your family, have an honest, open conversation about your health and the changes you're trying to make. You may want to recruit a friend or loved one into being your exercise partner. Involving your loved ones can be fun and can also bring additional closeness to your relationships.

There are also several support groups and organizations that can help you as you make changes. If you are looking to lose weight, you might want to investigate organizations like Overeaters Anonymous or Weight Watchers. If you want to reduce stress in your life, talk to someone at your local YMCA. They may be able to set up an exercise program for you, or recommend meditation or support groups that can help you work on specific issues of interest. Your doctor, dietitian, or health educator can also be valuable by guiding you to organizations and programs in your area that can offer additional support.

A WORD ON MODERATION

Remember: When it comes to making lifestyle changes, patience is indeed a virtue; regaining good health happens gradually. The lifestyle changes that we've discussed here may sometimes seem overwhelming or close to impossible. So take it easy, but take it. If you love red meat and can't imagine giving it up, don't go cold turkey. Instead, just don't eat it as often. Take it slow. You're not alone; thousands of black men just like you are grappling with the very same health issues. Find them. And look to your friends, family, physician, and this book for support. Ultimately, of course, the strength to change your lifestyle must come from within. But you're not alone.

Good luck as you go forward. You can do it!

And don't forget: Be aware of your body's red light warning signals. When you experience any new symptom, it may be a warning sign of a serious illness. By getting it treated immediately, or at least, early, you might avoid disabilities, such as a stroke, heart attack, loss of a limb, or even death. Notify your doctor and use reference books such as *Your Body's Red Light Warning System*, by Neil Shulman, M. D.; Jack Birge, M. D.; and Joon Ahn, M. D. (Dell, $5.99).

THREE

High Blood Pressure: The Silent Killer

NED'S STORY

High blood pressure can strike even the most unlikely candidates. Take Ned, for example. He was caught completely off guard when his professor diagnosed him with hypertension during a health administration class. Ned was 48 years old, well educated, and conscientious about his health and appearance. He weighed just over 200 pounds, and the weight was well distributed over his six-foot frame. In other ways, too, Ned had it made. In addition to being a handsome man with a good physique, he had a good job and a great wife, Sharon, who supported him in everything he did. The couple had two sons, ages 13 and 11, who gave them reasons to be proud.

Ned was a successful hospital administrator at a large inner-city hospital—in fact, the first black administrator the hospital had ever had. After working in that capacity for over a year, Ned had begun taking night classes, working toward his doctorate degree. Sharon supported her husband's decision to further his education although she saw less of him than usual and had to handle their two sons virtually alone.

One of Ned's assignments during his health administration course was to learn how to take blood pressure measurements. Ned, always willing, held up his hand when the professor asked for a volunteer. Besides, Ned was curious because he'd never paid much attention to blood pressure readings. The professor took Ned's blood pressure three times; each reading was well above normal. Ned was surprised and more than a bit concerned.

The professor advised Ned that, although his blood pressure wasn't dangerously high for a man his age, he should still have it checked by a doctor. Ned went home that night and told his wife about his blood pressure. She, too, was concerned, and they agreed Ned should see his doctor as soon as possible.

After Ned's doctor had run a few tests and asked several questions, he confirmed that Ned had high blood pressure. "But I don't feel sick," Ned said. "I feel great." The doctor explained that often people can have high blood pressure and not even know it. He also reassured the couple that high blood pressure is not a death sentence by any means. There are several things a person with high blood pressure can do to keep it under control. We'll talk about that later.

MONROE'S STORY

Monroe tends to better suit the typical high-blood-pressure profile: He was a large man, just as his father and grandfather had been, and about 30 pounds overweight. But his extra weight seemed part of his personality: He had a smile that could stop you on the street and pull you into his butcher shop for laughs and a pleasant break from the day's goings on.

Monroe's shop was the gathering place for people throughout the day. Monroe always had a pot of coffee on and a tray of sweets set out for the customers. At the end of his day, usually around six at night, Monroe would grab a few cuts of meat and head home. Monroe liked all aspects of food—from preparation to cooking and eating. He especially liked salty foods. Whenever he brought meat home from the shop, he would cook big, juicy steaks and then cover them with salt from the saltshaker. "You can never have enough salt," he used to say. "It improves the taste." Then he'd lick his lips jokingly. His wife used to tease him about it—it was an old joke between them. In fact, in their household, no meal was served without a saltshaker on the table.

One day, while Monroe was cutting ribs, he suddenly felt dizzy and weak. He set down his cleaver and leaned on the counter. The customer waiting for the ribs was concerned. "Monroe, you look pale," he said uneasily. After about 10 minutes, Monroe felt better and continued with the job at hand. That night, however, he told Cynthia about the incident. She asked him to go get a physical checkup; after all, it had been a couple of years since he had had one. At first, Monroe was against the idea, always picturing himself as a strong, healthy man. But his wife convinced him that getting the checkup was a good idea.

Doctors usually call high blood pressure "hypertension." (We'll use both terms interchangeably for this discussion.) It's also often called "the silent killer" because, as was true for Ned and Monroe, you can have high blood pressure without even knowing it. Often, it sneaks up slowly. Maybe, like Monroe, you've always enjoyed eating salty foods, and you're now paying the price. Maybe, like Ned, you're under a lot of stress. Or maybe, without knowing it, you are leading a lifestyle destined for tragedy. Destined for tragedy, that is, unless, of course, you're willing to make a change.

If you have high blood pressure, you should know that you aren't alone—it's a very common condition. Hypertension can be caused by your lifestyle, a predisposition in your genes, or both. If someone in your family had high blood pressure, keep a close eye on your own because you may be at increased risk. But whether you have been diagnosed with hypertension or not, it's important for you and your family to know how you can prevent and treat this disease.

WHAT IS HIGH BLOOD PRESSURE?

Blood pressure is the pressure of blood against the walls of your blood vessels—especially your arteries. Your heart pumps blood through your arteries with varying degrees of force. For example, certain types of exercises, such as lifting weights, cause your heart to pump harder and blood vessels to tighten, resulting in more pressure inside your blood vessels.[1]

There is a difference between hypertension, which is a health disorder, and occasional elevated blood pressure caused by normal physiological reactions. When you're participating in a strenuous activity or feeling emotional stress (such as the nervousness, tension, or anger brought on by a job interview, performance review, or argument), your blood pressure can rise. Do you remember ever being so frightened that you thought your heart would jump out of your chest? These incident-specific rises in blood pressure don't necessarily mean that you have high blood pressure or hypertension: Sure, your blood pressure measurement may be high during activities like these, but it quickly returns to normal once the events are over with. If you have high blood pressure or hypertension, on the other hand, your blood pressure stays constantly above what is considered normal.

WHY ARE BLACKS AT GREATER RISK?

Black males are 40 percent more likely to suffer from high blood pressure than white males, and usually develop more serious complications, such as kidney failure, as a result. Approximately 28 percent of all people on kidney dialysis machines are black although blacks make up only 12 percent of the population! High blood pressure kills black men about 15 times more often than it does white men, and one in three blacks has high blood pressure. Up to 30 percent of all deaths in hypertensive black men may be due to high blood pressure.[2] (Hypertension is more common among younger men than younger women; however, in middle age, more women than men have hypertension, perhaps because of the effects of menopause.)

Why are blacks more likely to suffer from high blood pressure than others? This question is tough to answer; indeed, the cause of 95 percent of all hypertension cases remains unknown. However, one characteristic that hypertensive patients seem to have in common is "too much"—too much salt in the diet, too much stress, too much weight, too much alcohol. High blood pressure may be caused by any one of these factors or a combination of several of them.

ESTIMATED PERCENTAGE OF AMERICANS WITH HIGH BLOOD PRESSURE BY SEX AND RACE: UNITED STATES 1988-94

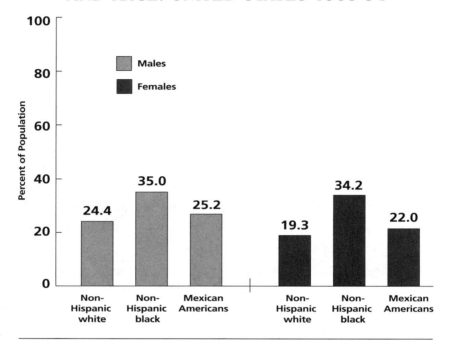

Reprinted from Center for Disease Control, "African Americans and Cardiovascular Diseases Biostatistical Fact Sheet" (NHANES III (1988-94), Health United States, 1988, CDC/NCHS.

DO BLACKS HAVE AN INHERITED KIDNEY DEFECT?

In one study, researchers suggested that blacks may have inherited a kidney defect that limits their ability to process sodium, an element found in salt. If this theory is correct, people with the kidney defect would not be properly able to handle salt already in their bodies, let alone any additional salt they add through diet.

If you have inherited this condition, even a small amount of salt in your food may cause your blood pressure to rise, putting you at a high risk for hypertension.[3]

DID IT REALLY ALL START WITH SLAVERY?

Dr. Clarence Grim of Drew Medical Center in Los Angeles offers another theory. When African natives were traded as slaves, the physical demands of the ocean voyage were very great. Many slaves died of dehydration, or loss of the water in their body tissues. Salt is necessary to hold water in your tissues. Therefore, according to Grim, only the best "salt savers" survived.

Although retaining fluid by saving salt was a boon on a voyage with little fresh water, the same characteristic can be harmful under normal conditions because it makes one more susceptible to high blood pressure. Since the tendency toward high blood pressure is often hereditary, Grim suggests that the first Americanized "salt savers" passed their strong tendency toward "salt saving" to future generations.[4] You can take this with a grain of salt!

CITY LIVING CAN LEAD TO HYPERTENSION

Several studies show that hypertension increases with the stress of urbanization. In 1984, Neil Poulter studied a tribe in Kenya that migrated to the city of Nairobi, measuring their blood pressures before and after the migration. Overall, the blood pressures increased. Later, the tribe was forced to flee the city. After the tribe members returned to a rural setting, Poulter saw that their blood pressures returned to their original low levels.

Ironically, our African ancestors were almost hypertension-free. However, as they moved away from their tribal villages to cities, high blood pressure became more common. This could be due to several factors, such as overcrowding, poverty, increased salt intake, poor eating habits leading to weight gain, or stress from political or racial discrimination. Whatever the reason, something has caused the blood pressure of us former Africans to rise.

DISCRIMINATION CAUSES STRESS

Some researchers, such as Michael Klag, whose study was published in the *Journal of the American Medical Association*, report that darker skin color itself can be a cause of stress that can lead to high blood pressure. Many dark black men who struggle daily to climb the socioeconomic ladder encounter complications because of racial barriers. These include stagnant job level and racism in the workplace. "Guilt by color" is a variety of that racism that you're probably familiar with. For example, when something goes wrong or winds up missing from the office, a black male may more likely be suspected and accused than his white co-workers. For the victim, this can be very frustrating, especially if it happens often. This constant level of frustration may contribute to high blood pressure.[5]

TWO TYPES OF HYPERTENSION

There are two types of hypertension. The first, known as "essential hypertension," accounts for approximately 95 percent of all high blood pressure cases. This term refers to those cases whose causes are unknown. Both Monroe and Ned were diagnosed with essential hypertension.

"Secondary hypertension" accounts for the other 5 percent of all high blood pressure cases. Secondary hypertension is caused by specific abnormalities such as some tumors, kidney disease, the blockage of certain arteries (such as kidney artery), or high levels of certain substances in your blood, such as cocaine. (Cocaine and crack have recently become established as common causes of secondary hypertension. For more information about drug and substance abuse, see Chapter 10.) Incidentally, when secondary hypertension has been caused by a tumor that releases an adrenaline-type substance, it can sometimes be corrected by surgery.

Now, let's take another look at Ned and Monroe.

NED AND MONROE REACT TO THEIR DIAGNOSES

Ned, upon learning of his condition, was anxious to know why he developed high blood pressure. He and his wife had decided to treat the disorder aggressively rather than sit back and let it run its course, so it was important to know its origin. They read all the latest studies and articles concerning high blood pressure, and talked to Ned's doctor extensively. Ned and his wife also looked into his family history to see if his high blood pressure could possibly be genetic.

They learned that some of Ned's family members were also living with the disease. "My uncle is an insurance broker," said Ned. "He travels a lot and eats out often. He knows better, but admits he doesn't watch his diet even though he takes his medicine regularly.

"Another cousin of mine didn't discover she had high blood pressure until she became pregnant," Ned continued. "The doctors watched her carefully during the delivery, and she has been on medication ever since. She's very careful about her diet."

But Ned and Sharon also learned, by looking at their own diets, that Ned regularly consumed too much sodium (found primarily in salt), a factor that can contribute heavily to the development of the disease.

When Monroe visited his doctor, he learned that his blood pressure was at a dangerous level. After answering a lot of questions, Monroe discovered that his lifestyle fit the classic profile of a hypertension candidate. Several factors had contributed to his high blood pressure: heredity for one. Like Ned, Monroe had a family history of high blood pressure. Of all the factors, however, Monroe's diet was probably the biggest contributor to his condition.

Monroe admitted to his doctor that he had a habit of always salting his food before he even tasted it. In addition, Monroe had many bad eating habits, such as his love of red meat and peanuts. Because he had been eating fat-filled foods like these throughout his entire life, Monroe learned he was also a high-risk candidate for heart disease (see Chapter 4).

The doctor talked to Monroe and Cynthia for a long time, explaining the benefits of good diet and exercise. Monroe never was one to exercise, preferring to spend his spare time in long conversations with customers. The couple listened to the doctor intently and, upon leaving the office, stopped by their local pharmacy to fill Monroe's new prescription. Monroe took his medicine for hypertension every day, but was unwilling to change his diet. Cynthia tried to convince her husband to eat more healthy foods, without success.

HOW CAN I PREVENT HIGH BLOOD PRESSURE?

In Chapter 2, we discussed many ways to prevent disease. Although no studies have proved a single cause of essential hypertension, researchers have discovered several ways to keep this condition from developing into more serious consequences like heart attack or stroke.

- *Limit salt in your diet*
  Studies show that too much salt in the diet is closely associated with hypertension. To prevent and treat high blood pressure, it's important to reduce your salt intake. For more information about salty foods to avoid and how to improve your diet generally, see Chapter 2.

- *Reduce stress*
  A number of different factors have been associated with high blood pressure—stress is one. Like Ned, many of us lead active, hectic lives. Though we may find our busy lives fulfilling, by constantly putting ourselves in situations that make us tense, we put great pressure on our circulatory systems. We should all make a conscious effort to reduce our stress levels, especially if someone in our family has already had high blood pressure because that alone could put us at increased risk. (More information about stress reduction is included in Chapter 2.)

- *Increase your potassium intake*
  When it comes to preventing hypertension, it's also important to make sure you're getting enough potassium in your diet since research shows a link between low potassium

intake and high blood pressure. Many studies show that blacks in the United States consume less potassium than whites. One reason for this may be that, overall, blacks eat less fresh fruit than whites, and both fresh fruits and vegetables contain high levels of potassium. Further, remember, if you overcook vegetables, you lose much of the potassium and vitamins that these foods offer. Finally, if you choose prune juice as a source of potassium, realize that prunes are also a laxative. If you notice your stools getting loose, choose another potassium source instead.

Try to increase your intake of potassium naturally through foods, if you can. Just don't overdo it. No study has proved that taking potassium supplements will necessarily lower your blood pressure, so get your doctor's approval before taking this route. As in most things, moderation is the rule here: High potassium levels can be dangerous if you have an illness such as kidney disease, so you'll want to be especially careful if this pertains to you.

- *Increase your calcium intake*
  Some researchers have also suggested that low levels of calcium in the diet may contribute to hypertension. However, this is still under debate.

- *Avoid licorice and chewing tobacco*
  In some cases, licorice and chewing tobacco can cause high blood pressure because these substances may contain a steroid-like compound that stimulates your kidneys to hold on to sodium. This compound also causes your body to hold onto fluids, which can elevate your blood pressure. So if you're prone to high blood pressure, it's best to avoid both licorice and chewing tobacco.[6] (Since chewing tobacco has

POTASSIUM-RICH FOODS

Item	Amount	Milliequivalents of Potassium	Calories	Milligrams of Sodium
Prune juice*	1 glass+	15.1	193	5
Tomato juice	1 glass	13.7	48	480
Cantaloupe	One-half	12.8	60	24
Potato (baked)	One medium	12.8	95	4
Grapefruit juice	1 glass	11.8	108	3
Orange juice	1 glass	10.7	120	3
Milk (skim)	1 glass	10.5	89	128
Raisins	1/3 cup	10.4	153	14
Milk (whole)	1 glass	9.5	150	120
Banana	One 6"	9.5	85	1
Pineapple juice	1 glass	9.2	128	<1
Tomato	One medium	8.1	29	5
Orange	One medium	8.0	71	2
Pear	One medium	6.7	122	4
Apple juice	1 glass	6.2	120	8
Peach	One medium	5.2	38	1
Apple	One medium	4.2	87	1
Grapefruit	One-half	3.5	41	1
Black coffee	1 cup	2.2	2	1

* All juice values are as canned, unsweetened.
+ 1 glass = 8 ounces.

Note: The recommended daily limit for sodium intake is less than 2,400 milligrams for people with high blood pressure.

SELECTED CALCIUM-RICH FOOD SOURCES

Dairy foods	mg calcium
Buttermilk, 1 cup	285
Cheese, American, 1 oz.	174
Cheese, Cheddar, 1 oz.	204
Cheese, ricotta, part skim, 4 oz.	308
Cheese, Swiss, 1 oz.	272
Ice cream, vanilla, _ cup	84
Milk, whole, 1 cup	291
Milk, 2%, 1 cup	297
Milk, skim, 1 cup	302
Yogurt, fruit, lowfat, 1 cup	383
Yogurt, plain, skim, 1 cup	488

Beans/seafood	
Baked beans, plain or vegetarian, 1 cup	127
Salmon, canned with bones, 3 oz.	181
Sardines, with bones, 3 oz.	325

Vegetables	
Beet greens, boiled, _ cup	82
Bok choy, boiled, _ cup	79
Broccoli, stalk, raw,	155
Collards, frozen, boiled, _ cup	179
Kale, frozen, boiled, _ cup	89
Mustard greens, frozen, boiled, _ cup	76
Spinach, boiled, _ cup	122

Grains	
Corn bread, from recipe with 2% milk, 1 piece	162
Pancakes, from recipe, 4-inch diameter, 2	166
Waffles, from recipe, 7-inch diameter, 1	191

Source: USDA Nutrient Database for Standard Reference.

been linked to increased risk of oral cancer, it's a good idea to avoid this anyway.)

- *Prevent and treat obesity*
  Excess weight puts a strain on your heart as well as your body. High blood pressure is more common in obese people than in people with normal body weight. If you know you're prone to high blood pressure, it would be especially wise for you to maintain the ideal weight for your height and body frame. If you think you should lose weight, consult your doctor. Then, reread Chapter 2 for tips on how to begin.

HOW DO I KNOW IF I HAVE HYPERTENSION?

If you experience sudden temporary blindness, chest pain, dizziness, or severe pounding headaches, see a doctor immediately since these can be symptoms of severe high blood pressure. Nosebleeds, though common among people with normal blood pressure levels, can also be a sign of dangerously high blood pressure. If you're experiencing any of these symptoms, get your blood pressure checked immediately.

Even if you're not experiencing these symptoms, it's still important to monitor your blood pressure regularly. Remember that high blood pressure can be a silent killer. That's why many people, like Ned, aren't aware they have high blood pressure. If left undetected and untreated, hypertension can surprise you in the form of a heart attack, stroke, kidney failure, or blindness. (See Chapter 4 for more information about heart disease.) To find out if you need to take precautions against these tragedies, have a health professional check your blood pressure regularly. Or you can check it yourself.

HOW BLOOD PRESSURE IS MEASURED

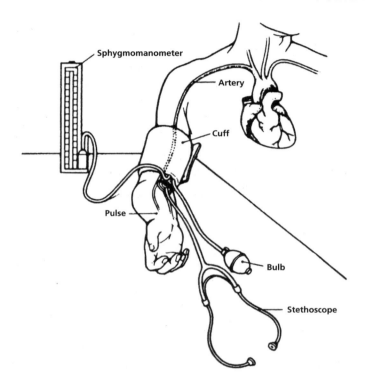

TAKING YOUR BLOOD PRESSURE

You have two options: You can take your own blood pressure or have someone else take it for you. If you decide to take it yourself, you need a blood pressure kit. The kit will contain an arm cuff with a pressure gauge attached to it (sphygmomanometer) and a listening device (stethoscope). You'll need to purchase a cuff that is the correct width for your arm: Large widths are necessary if the circumference of your upper arm is more than 13 inches. You can purchase these kits at most pharmacies for about $30. You can also purchase a more expensive, electronic blood pressure kit that, instead of a stethoscope, uses a digital display.

Before you take your blood pressure, make sure you are relaxed and have been sitting down for at least five minutes. Then:

1. Locate your pulse in the bend of your elbow with your finger.

2. Wrap the cuff around your upper arm, leaving about 1 inch between the bottom of the cuff and the bend of your elbow. Be sure that nothing is caught under the cuff, such as your clothing, since this may affect the reading.

3. Hold the rubber bulb so that the screw lies between your thumb and forefinger. Inflate the cuff by squeezing the rubber bulb until you can no longer feel your pulse beat in your wrist. Write down the number on the gauge at this point.

4. Turn the screw toward you (to the left), releasing the pressure out of the cuff until the gauge reads zero.

5. Add 30 to the first number you wrote down and pump up the cuff until the gauge reads this number.

6. Place the stethoscope directly over the main artery of your arm (brachial artery).

7. Slowly releasing the air on the gauge, listen for the first tapping sound. When you hear it, note the number on the gauge. This is the systolic pressure, the top number of your blood pressure reading.

8. The number on the gauge at the last sound or tapping noise you hear is the diastolic pressure, the bottom number of your blood pressure.[7]

If you have a hearing impairment, you may not be able to hear the tapping sounds through the stethoscope. Your doctor or a nurse should be able to instruct you in your blood pressure measurement and verify the accuracy of your equipment by checking your readings with his or her own.

WHAT HAPPENS WHEN MY BLOOD PRESSURE IS TAKEN?

When the cuff is wrapped around your upper arm and inflated, the air pressure in the cuff pushes against the main artery of your arm and nearby bone. This stops your flow of blood. When the pressure is released, your blood flows freely again, making a "whooshing" sound through the narrowed artery. The number on the gauge when this sound is made is the systolic pressure. A normal blood pressure reading is less than 130/85 (a new report says that for middle aged men the figure is 140/90 or less0. The top number is the systolic pressure measurement and the bottom number represents the diastolic measurement. When your blood flow finally evens out and your blood vessel is no longer narrowed, the sound disappears. The number on the gauge at the last sound you will hear will be the diastolic pressure. Except in extreme cases, the lower your blood pressure is, the better off you are. The higher your blood pressure, the greater risk you run of complications. This is true for both the top (systolic) and the bottom (diastolic) number.

If you decide to have someone else take your blood pressure, you have several options. Any medical professional, including health clinic employees, nurses, health educators, doctors, dentists, and pharmacists, should be able to take your blood pressure

CLASSIFICATION OF BLOOD PRESSURE
FOR ADULTS AGE 18 YEARS AND OLDER*

Category	Systolic (mm Hg)	Diastolic (mm Hg)
Optimal	<120	<80
Normal**	<130	<85
High normal	130–139	85–89
Hypertension***		
Stage 1	140–159	90–99
Stage 2	160–179	100–109
Stage 3	>180	>110

* The figures apply to people who are not taking antihypertensive drugs and not acutely ill. When systolic and diastolic pressures fall into different categories, the higher category should be selected to classify the individual's blood pressure status. For instance, 160/92 mm Hg should be classified as Stage 2, and 180/120 mm Hg should be classified as Stage 3. Isolated systolic hypertension (ISH) is defined as SBP≥140 mm Hg and DBP <90 mm Hg, and staged appropriately (e.g., 170/85 mm Hg is defined as Stage 2 ISH).

** Optimal blood pressure with respect to cardiovascular risk is SBP<120 mm Hg and DBP <80 mm Hg. However, unusually low readings should be evaluated for clinical significance.

*** Based on the average of two or more readings taken at each of two or more visits following an initial screening.

Note: In addition to classifying stages of hypertension based on average blood pressure levels, the clinician should specify presence or absence of target-organ—that is, brain, eyes, heart, or kidney—disease and additional risk factors. For example, a patient with diabetes and blood pressure of 142/94 mm Hg plus an enlarged left heart muscle (left ventricular hypertrophy) should be classified as "Stage 1 hypertension with target-organ disease (left ventricular hypertrophy) and with another major risk factor (diabetes)." This specificity is important for risk classification and management.

Reprinted from the *Sixth Report of the Joint National Committee on Prevention, Detection, Evaluation, and Treatment of High Blood Pressure,* from the National institute of Health, Heart, Lung, and Blood Institute. NIH publication No. 98–4080, November 1997.

reading. It's always a good idea to have your blood pressure measured whenever you visit a medical professional, even if you're there for another reason. Let your doctor or health care professional know that you would like your blood pressure checked regularly; they can help you find an inexpensive—or even free—way to keep your pressure checked regularly.

How often should you have your blood pressure checked? If your pressure is within the normal range (less than 130/85), it's safe to have it checked every other year until you reach age 40. If you are older than 40 and/or your blood pressure is higher than 130/85, you should have your blood pressure checked twice a year.

NED, MONROE, AND STRESS

When Ned reflected on his lifestyle, it was clear that stress was a cause of his high blood pressure. It was also clear that this stress came from his job and from the additional new pressure of taking night classes after work. His job as hospital administrator, though the prestige was gratifying, required him to work long hours to keep up with the mountain of paperwork that gathered on his desk weekly.

Even today, against his wife's wishes, he sometimes still works weekends. According to his wife, he always says, "If I work late this one night, I'll be caught up," or "Just this one weekend and then never again." Ned admits the workload has, indeed, been heavy. And he pays a heavy price—in the form of frequent headaches, loss of appetite, and sleeplessness.

Ned's job was too important to him for him to give it up. But eventually, with Sharon's help, Ned learned to alleviate stress buildup through exercise.

"Sharon and I don't have all the answers," said Ned. "But we're

both determined to do everything possible to keep my disease under control. It helps when you have support from your family. This isn't something you can do alone. The fact that I feel better and handle the stress better, even though I can't get rid of it, makes Sharon happy, too. Not only am I healthier, but she says I'm more fun to be with."

MONROE'S EATING HABITS

In Monroe's search for the cause of his high blood pressure, stress was not at the top of the list. In his case, diet and obesity were the number-one and number-two risk factors.

Although Monroe knew his eating habits weren't healthy, he wasn't willing to change them. Cynthia tried to keep an eye on him, but she couldn't be with him every minute of every day. At home, much to his dismay, she took over cooking to ensure that he ate healthy foods. She even let him cook an occasional steak, but she tried to center meals on baked or broiled chicken and fish. She refused to use salt when cooking, substituting a variety of spices and seasonings instead.

When Monroe was on his own, the only thing he did right was take his medicine. Since his wife wouldn't let him eat salty food at home, he started going to fast-food restaurants every day for lunch. Because he wasn't willing to take control of his own health, he began gaining even more weight.

WHAT CAN HAPPEN IF I DON'T TREAT MY HYPERTENSION?

If you've been diagnosed with high blood pressure and, like Monroe, decide not to make important lifestyle changes, the consequences can be deadly:

- *Your risk of having a stroke increases*
  Left untreated, high blood pressure can cause strokes. Though
  the exact reason for this is not known, it seems that high
  blood pressure injures your arterial walls and allows plaques
  (fat and cholesterol buildup) to attach to the scarring. When
  high blood pressure goes unchecked, it can sometimes cause
  enough buildup of fatty deposits and pressure to block your
  arteries completely. When this blockage occurs in an artery
  that supplies your brain with blood, a stroke may occur. (We
  discuss strokes further in Chapter 4.) According to the Office
  of Minority Health, blacks have strokes twice as often as
  whites. Not only that, but black men are also almost twice as
  likely to die from stroke as white men.

- *You're at greater risk of kidney disease*
  Uncontrolled high blood pressure can also damage your kidneys. The kidneys' inability to rid your body of wastes
  becomes impaired, which can result in a whole host of diseases
  and disorders related to kidney malfunction. See Chapter 8 for
  more detailed information on kidney or renal failure.

- *You may develop heart disease*
  High blood pressure contributes to heart disease. As the
  amount of pressure increases in your arteries, your heart has
  to work harder to circulate blood throughout your body.
  The harder your heart works, the more your heart muscle
  builds and enlarges, making it less efficient. Further, the
  coronary arteries that supply blood to your heart may
  become blocked, resulting in death of heart tissue (heart
  attack). For more detailed information on heart disease, see
  Chapter 4.

COMPLICATIONS OF HIGH BLOOD PRESSURE

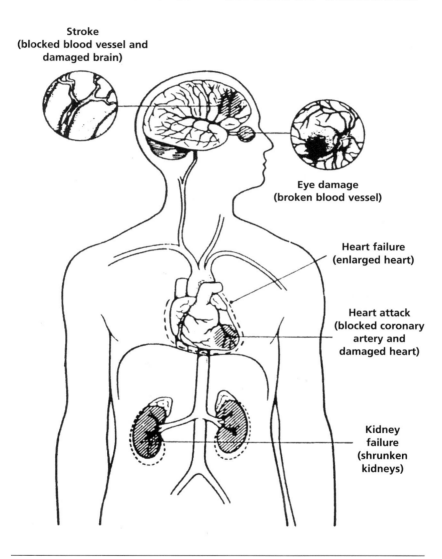

Stroke
(blocked blood vessel and
damaged brain)

Eye damage
(broken blood vessel)

Heart failure
(enlarged heart)

Heart attack
(blocked coronary
artery and
damaged heart)

Kidney
failure
(shrunken
kidneys)

Reprinted with permission of authors from High Blood Pressure by Neil Shulman, Elijah Saunders, and W. Dallas Hall, copyright 1987 by Neil Shulman, M.D., Elijah Saunders, M.D., and W. Dallas Hall, M.D.

HOW CAN I TREAT MY HIGH BLOOD PRESSURE?

Unfortunately, black males are notorious for not seeking medical treatment and for not continuing it when it has been prescribed. Approximately 50 percent of black men with high blood pressure drop out of treatment in the first year. One-half of those who stay under medical care do not take their prescribed medicine regularly enough to achieve adequate blood pressure reduction. This may be one reason why relatively more black men than white men die of complications from high blood pressure.

To be sure, money can be a problem. Once you have high blood pressure, the cost can run $30 a month or more for medication to control high blood pressure. But if you let your blood pressure go untreated, dialysis to treat kidney failure can run around $45,000 a year. Put bluntly, you'll save yourself a lot of money—not to mention suffering—by controlling your blood pressure with medication. Like so many other health problems, high blood pressure can be a lifestyle issue. So here are some things you can do to help you avoid high blood pressure or to lower it once you get it:

- *Exercise*
  Exercise, exercise, exercise. Regular exercise improves circulation throughout your body and enhances your body's ability to use oxygen. Exercise also increases your energy level, reduces stress and tension, helps you lose weight, and makes it easier for you to relax and sleep.

  It is never too late to start an exercise program. Before you begin, ask your doctor for advice, especially if you have already been diagnosed with high blood pressure, because certain types of exercise, such as weightlifting, may be dangerous. For more information about how to begin your own personalized exercise program, see Chapter 2.

- *Limit your alcohol intake*
  If you're already hypertensive, alcohol consumption makes your disorder more difficult to control and can get in the way of blood pressure medication. Limit your alcohol intake. (Ideally, you should avoid it altogether.) However, if you choose to drink alcohol, use the rule of moderation. Try to limit your daily intake to no more than one or two drinks (one drink is equivalent to an 8-ounce glass of wine, a 12-ounce glass of beer, or a 1-ounce shot of hard liquor).

- *Take your high blood pressure medication*
  Your doctor will tell you which medications, if any, you should take if you're diagnosed with high blood pressure. But it is up to you to ask questions. Many high blood pressure medications can cause side effects. You and your doctor should choose those that will work best for you.

HYPERTENSION MEDICATION

When your doctor prescribes a new medication, ask him or her for free samples. That way, if you develop an unpleasant side effect, you have not wasted money by purchasing an entire prescription. Many hypertension medications are on the market today, so it's a good idea to make sure you are taking one that best suits your needs. Have your doctor explain to you the advantages and disadvantages of several. After all, once you have high blood pressure, you will usually have it for the rest of your life, and you'll need to continue taking medication, so you want to get the one best for you.

Impotence is one side effect that prevents some men from staying on blood pressure medication. But remember that impotence is a rare side effect of high blood pressure medication, and recent advances have been made in high blood pressure medication so that you can control your blood pressure without suffering impotence. To find out if impotence is a possible side effect of your medication, consult the list of high blood pressure medications in Figure 3G. If you think the medication you're taking is causing your impotence, ask your doctor about possibly changing your prescription.[8]

No matter what, don't stop taking your high blood pressure medication without your doctor's consent, even if you're feeling great. Remember, hypertension is a silent killer.

REMEMBERING TO TAKE YOUR MEDICATION

So you're forgetful? Afraid you can't remember to take your pills? Here are some suggestions that may help you.

- Place your pills or capsules where you will notice them when doing a daily task, such as brushing your teeth.

- Keep your pills in separate containers that are labeled with the time you should take them, such as at breakfast, lunch, dinner, or bedtime.

- Wear a watch with an alarm that rings when you need to take your medication.

- Mark your calendar every time you take your medicine.

- At the beginning of each day, set out the pills you'll need to take.

- Keep extra pills handy, in case you run out before your next visit to the doctor.

- If you are going out for the day, or on vacation, remember to pack/take your medication with you.

NED, MONROE, AND EXERCISE

Ned isn't overweight, but he now exercises several days a week, sometimes with Sharon, sometimes by himself. He runs three days a week—sometimes before work and sometimes after, depending on his schedule. He also plays basketball with his friends at least twice a week. He says that the activity seems to reduce his stress and makes him feel better. "It's a lot easier to face the day after a vigorous walk or jog," Ned said. "I also find that running after work is a good time to reflect on my day. Sure, exercise takes some time, but what keeps me alive and well is time well spent."

Monroe's story took a different turn. The exercise program suggested by his doctor never got farther than the walk to the bakery.

CONCLUSION

Don't let yourself become a victim of your condition, like Monroe. If you were able to identify with any of the risks mentioned in this chapter, act now. Although black males seem to be more prone to hypertension than other people, you don't have to become the next

ORAL ANTIHYPERTENSIVE DRUGS AND THEIR SIDE-EFFECTS

Drug	Trade Name	Usual Dose Range, Total mg/day* (Frequency per Day)	Selected Side Effects and Comments*
DIURETICS (PARTIAL LIST)			
			Short-term: increase cholesterol and glucose levels; biochemical abnormalities: decreases potassium, sodium, and magnesium levels, increases uric acid and calcium levels; rare: blood dyscrasias, photosensitivity, pancreatitis, hyponatremia
Chlorthalidone (G)†	Hygroton	12.5–50 (1)	
Hydrochlorothiazide (G)	Hydrodiuril, Esidrix	12.5–50 (1)	
Indapamide	Lozol	1.25–5 (1)	(Less or no hypercholesterolemia)
Metrolazone	Mykrox	0.5–1.0 (1)	
	Zaroxolyn	2.5–10 (1)	
Loop diuretics			
Bumetanide (G)	Bumex	0.5–4 (2–3)	(Short duration of action, no hypercalcemia)
Ethacrynic acid	Edecrin	25–100 (2–3)	Only nonsulfonamide diuretic, ototoxicity)
Furosemide (G)	Lasix	40–240 (2–3)	(Short duration of action, no hypercalcemia)
Torsemide	Demadex	5–100 (1–2)	
Potassium-sparing agents			
Amiloride hydrochloride (G)	Midamor	5–10 (1)	
Spironolactone (G)	Aldactone	25–100 (1)	(Gynecomastia)
Triamterene (G)	Dyrenium	25–200 (1)	
ADRENERGIC INHIBITORS			
Peripheral agents			
Guanadrel	Hylorel	10–75 (2)	(Postural hypotension, diarrhea)
Guanethidine monosulfate	Ismelin	10–150 (1)	(Postural hypotension, diarrhea)

Drug	Trade Name	Usual Dose Range, Total mg/day* (Frequency per Day)	Selected Side Effects and Comments*
Reserpine (G)**	Serpasil	0.05–0.25 (1)	(Nasal congestion, sedation, depression, activation of peptic ulcer) Sedation, dry mouth, bradycardia, withdrawal hypertension

Central alpha-agonists

Drug	Trade Name	Dose	Comments
Clonidine hydrochloride (G)	Catapres	0.2–1.2 (2–3)	(More withdrawal)
Guanabenz acetate (G)	Wytensin	8–32 (2)	
Guanfacine hydrochloride (G)	Tenex	1–3 (1)	(Less withdrawal)
Methyldopa (G)	Aldomet	500–3,000 (2)	(Hepatic and "autoimmune" disorders)

Alpha-blockers

Drug	Trade Name	Dose	
Doxazosin mesylate	Cardura	1–16 (1)	
Prazosin hydrochloride (G)	Minipress	2–30 (2–3)	
Terazosin hydrochloride	Hytrin	1–20 (1)	

Beta-blockers

Drug	Trade Name	Dose	Comments
			Bronchospasm, bradycardia, heart failure, may mask insulin-induced hypoglycemia; less serious: impaired peripheral circulation, insomnia, fatigue, decreased exercise tolerance, hypertriglyceridemia (except agents with intrinsic sympathomimetric activity)
Acebutolol§‡	Sectral	200–800 (1)	
Atenolol (G)§	Tenormin	25–100 (1–2)	
Betaxolol§	Kerlone	5–20 (1)	
Bisoprolol fumarate§	Zebeta	2.5–10 (1)	
Carteolol hydrochloride‡	Cartrol	2.5–10 (1)	
Metoprolol tartrate (G)§	Lopressor	50–300 (2)	
Metoprolol succinate§	Toprol-XL	50–300 (1)	
Nadolol (G)	Corgard	40–320 (1)	
Penbutolol sulfate‡	Levatol	10–20 (1)	
Pindolol (G)‡	Visken	10–60 (2)	

continued on the next page

"Oral Hypertensive Drugs and Their Side Effects," continued

Drug	Trade Name	Usual Dose Range, Total mg/day* (Frequency per Day)	Selected Side Effects and Comments*
Propranolol hydrochloride (G)	Inderal Inderal LA	40–480 (1) 40–480 (2	
Timolol maleate (G)	Blocadren	20–60 (2)	
Combined alpha- and beta-blockers			Postural hypotension, bronchospasm
Carvedilol	Coreg	12.5–50 (2)	
Labetalol hydrochloride (G)	Normodyne, Trandate	200–1,200 (2)	

DIRECT VASODILATORS

Drug	Trade Name	Usual Dose Range	Selected Side Effects
Hydralazine hydrochloride (G)	Apresoline	50–300 (2)	(Lupus syndrome)
Minoxidil (G)	Loniten	5–100 (1)	(Hirsutism)

CALCIUM ANTAGONISTS

Nondihydropyridines

Drug	Trade Name	Usual Dose Range	Selected Side Effects
Diltiazem hydrochloride	Cardizem SR Cardizem CD, Dilacor XR, Tiazac	120–360 (2) 120–360 (1)	(Nausea, headache)
Mibefradil dihydrochloride (T-channel calcium antagonist)	Posicor	50–100 (1)	(No worsening of systolic dysfunction,' contraindicated with terfenadine [Seldane], astemizole [Hismanal], and cisapride [Propulsid])
Verapamil hydrochloride	Isoptin SR, Calan SR Verelan, Covera HS	90–480 (2) 120–480 (1)	(Constipation)

Dihydropyridines

Edema of the ankle, flushing, headache, gingival hypertrophy

Drug	Trade Name	Usual Dose Range	
Amlodipine besylate	Norvasc	2.5–10 (1)	
Felodipine	Plendil	2.5–20 (1)	
Isradipine	DynaCirc DynaCirc CR	5–20 (2) 5–20 (1)	
Nicardipine	Cardene SR	60–90 (2)	

Drug	Trade Name	Usual Dose Range, Total mg/day* (Frequency per Day)	Selected Side Effects and Comments*
Nifedipine	Procardia XL, Adalat CC	30–120 (1)	
Nisoldipine	Sular	20–60 (1)	

ACE INHIBITORS

			Common: cough; rare: angioedema, hyperkalemia, rash, loss of taste, leukopenia
Benazerpil hydrochloride	Lotensin	5–40 (1–2)	
Captopril (G)	Capoten	25–150 (2–3)	
Enalapril maleate	Vasotec	5–40 (1–2)	
Fosinopril sodium	Monopril	10–40 (1–2)	
Lisinopril	Prinivil, Zestril	5–40 (1)	
Moexipril	Univasc	7.5–15 (2)	
Quinarpil hydrochloride	Accupril	5–80 (1–2)	
Ramipril	Altace	1.25–20 (1–2)	
Trandolapril	Mavik	1–4 (1)	

ANGIOTENSIN II RECEPTOR BLOCKERS

			Angioedema (very rare), hyperkalemia
Losartan potassium	Cozaar	25–100 (1–2)	
Valsartan	Diovan	80–320 (1)	
Irbesartan	Avapro	150–300 (1)	

* These dosages may vary from those listed in the *Physicians' Desk Reference* (51st edition), which may be consulted for additional information. The listing of side effects is not all-inclusive, and side effects are for the class of drugs where noted for individual drugs (in parenthesis); clinicians are urged to refer to the package insert for a more detailed listing.
† (G) indicated generic available.
‡ Has iintrinsic sympathomimetic activity.
§ Cardioselective.
** Also acts centrally.

Reprinted from JNC VI.

statistic. Take a long, hard look at your lifestyle. It is never too late to learn from stories like those of Ned and Monroe.

The fact is, Monroe's health continues to fail. Although he still takes his medication, he takes no responsibility for his treatment, and remains a victim of his high blood pressure.

Ned, on the other hand, took an aggressive attitude toward controlling his high blood pressure. As a result, today he enjoys a healthy lifestyle. The only reminder he has of his condition is his high blood pressure medicine, which he takes every day. Because he was willing to make changes in his lifestyle, Ned has found new levels of fulfillment by taking personal responsibility for his own health and relying on his family and friends for support.

RESOURCES

American Red Cross
431 18th Street
Washington, DC 20006
(202) 639-3520
http://www.redcross.org
(Contact your local chapter for services provided by the American Red Cross related to high blood pressure.)

National Heart, Lung, and Blood Institute
NHLBI Information Center
P.O. Box 30105
Bethesda, MD 20824-0105
(301) 592-8573
http://www.nhlbi.nih.gov
Heart Health Toll-Free Information Line:
800-575-WELL (9355)

(The Center offers publications on heart disease, high blood pressure, and other topics.)

International Society on Hypertension in Blacks
2045 Manchester Street, N.E.
Atlanta, GA 30324-4110
(404) 875-6263
(The Society provides materials on conferences, workshops, and research, as well as patient education brochures. Membership is available.)

National Kidney Foundation
30 East 33rd Street
New York, NY 10016
(212) 889-2210
(800) 622-9010
http://www.kidney.org
(The Foundation provides a catalog that lists available educational materials.)

U.S. Pharmacopoeial Convention, Inc.
12601 Twinbrook Parkway
Rockville, MD 20852
(301) 881-0666
(800) 822-8772
http://www.usp.org
(The Convention's website offers answers to many frequently asked medication questions.)

NOTES FOR CHAPTER 3

1. Shulman, Neil B., Saunders, Elijah, and Hall, W. Dallas (1987), *High Blood Pressure*, New York, Macmillan Publishing Company, pp. 2–3.
2. African Americans and Cardiovascular Diseases, *Biostatistical Fact Sheets*, 1996, American Heart Association.
3. Hall, W. Dallas, Saunders, Elijah, and Shulman, Neil B. (1985), *Hypertension in Blacks: Epidemiology, Pathophysiology and Treatment*, Year Book Medical Publishers, Inc., Chicago, pp. 106–112.
4. Greenberg, Joel, "Science/Medicine," *Los Angeles Times*, September 30, 1991, p. B3.
5. Klag, Michael (1991), "Association of Skin Color and Blood Pressure vs. Blacks with Low Socio-Economic Status," *JAMA*, vol. 265, pp. 599–602.
6. Shulman, Saunders, and Hall, *High Blood Pressure*, p. 45.
7. Ibid., pp. 14–15.
8. Ibid., pp. 85–86.

FOUR

Heart Disease and Stroke

SECTION ONE: HEART DISEASE
CLAUDE'S STORY

Heart disease can go with inactivity. For many people, years of sitting on the couch have helped them pack on the pounds—one of the risk factors for heart disease. The fact is, however, that even the most active people can be caught unaware. Here's what happened to Claude.

Ever since he retired from the Marines after 30 years of service and several tours of duty, Claude has doted on this garden. His wife loves it because it keeps her busy canning, and they are never at a loss for vegetables. His neighbors love it because it's not unusual for them to wake up on Saturday morning and find grocery bags full of tomatoes, cucumbers, squash, and corn sitting on their front porches.

If you had to describe Claude in one word, that word would be "physical." He stayed in great shape while in the Marines, always passing his physical exams with flying colors. Even at age 59, Claude spends mornings walking through his garden, weeding, picking, or planting. He rests in the afternoons with a good book. Then in the

77

early evening, he and his wife often take a long walk. He also goes to his doctor for regular checkups. His steady good health was one reason it took Claude so long to take his occasional chest pains seriously. His only problems seem to be slightly elevated blood pressure and cholesterol levels.

WHAT IS HEART DISEASE?

Cardiovascular disease (sometimes just called "heart disease") is the leading killer of Americans, including African American men, and accounted for 33.8 percent of all deaths among African American men in 1997.[1] Cardiovascular disease includes high blood pressure, coronary heart disease (heart attack and chest pain called angina pectoris), stroke, and rheumatic fever and rheumatic heart disease. And even though you, like Claude, may think you are in good health, you may be at risk for heart disease without even knowing it.

As you read this page, your heart is pumping blood throughout your body approximately 80 times per minute—that's over 115,000 times in one day or more than 40 million times each year. To prevent heart disease, it is important to take precautions every day, whether you're healthy or not. (See Chapter 2 for more information about this.) Because it is a large muscle, your heart needs lots of nourishment to keep up its pace. Anything you put into your body that clogs your coronary arteries (straw-sized vessels on the surface of and within the heart muscle) can make your heart's job more difficult and eventually cause health problems. When something goes wrong that blocks or decreases the amount of blood that nourishes the heart itself, problems can occur.

Your heart is a strong muscle that lies behind your breast-bone in the left center of your chest. It serves as a pump with four rooms or chambers, two on top and two on the bottom. Each upper chamber is known as an atrium, the lower chambers as ventricles. Your upper chambers receive blood from your veins and serve as reservoirs. The lower chambers, ventricles, are the pumping chambers of your heart. Here's how it works: The right atrium receives blood from the veins of the body. The blood then enters the right ventricle where it is pumped to the lungs, where the blood receives a fresh supply of oxygen. Then the oxygen-containing (oxygenated) blood passes to the left atrium, delivered to the left ventricle where it is then pumped out to the body.

Your blood goes from one chamber to another and out of your heart through four valves, which act like one-way doors, let-ting blood flow through them in only one direction. Each valve has two or three flaps, the cusps, which open and close with the force of the blood in your heart. The two valves between your atria and ventricles are called the mitral valve and the tricuspid valve. The aortic valve opens to let blood flow out of your left ventricle and into your aorta (the main vessel supplying blood to your body). The pulmonary valve allows blood to flow out of your right ventricle to your lungs through the pulmonary artery (the main blood vessel supplying blood to your lungs).

Now that you know the basics of how your heart functions, let's talk about the four major problems that can affect it:

1. Your coronary arteries (blood vessels supplying the heart) can get clogged.

2. Your heart muscle can weaken.

3. The valves within your heart can get stuck or not open properly.

4. You can develop a disorder of the electrical impulses of your heart, which can result in irregular heart rhythms. (To learn more about heart rhythms, see the section on arrhythmias on page 93.)

CROSS SECTION OF THE HEART

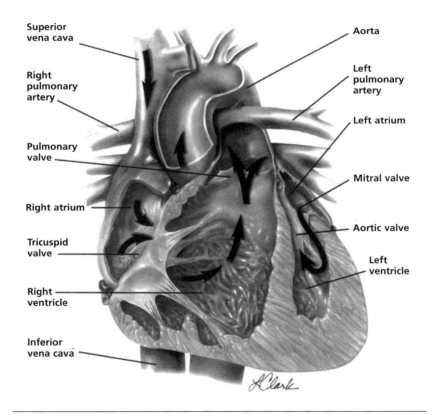

Superior vena cava

Right pulmonary artery

Pulmonary valve

Right atrium

Tricuspid valve

Right ventricle

Inferior vena cava

Aorta

Left pulmonary artery

Left atrium

Mitral valve

Aortic valve

Left ventricle

Reprinted with permission of the American Heart Association, "Heart and Stroke Facts" (1999), p. 3.

CLAUDE LISTENS TO REASON

The first time the pain occurred, Claude was tilling his garden, preparing it for winter. The pain started in his chest and radiated out toward his arms and jaw. Experiencing difficulty in breathing, Claude shut down the tiller and sat down in the shade. Within 10 to 15 minutes, he felt better. He put away the tiller and finished the job later in the week. The next time the pain came, he was carrying bags of fertilizer to the shed. Again, Claude stopped what he was doing, rested a while and soon felt better. The third time occurred during one of his evening walks with his wife. She was concerned and asked him to make an appointment to see his doctor. By this time, Claude was worried enough to agree.

When Claude described his attacks of pain, his doctor had a good idea what was wrong, but to be certain, he ordered a battery of tests. Sure enough, Claude had been experiencing "angina pectoris" attacks—chest pain that occurs when there's not enough blood flowing to nourish the heart muscle. The doctor explained to Claude that a combination of his age and high blood pressure had contributed to the condition. After running a battery of specific tests, the doctor suggested that, for the time being at least, Claude needed only to take nitroglycerin medication when he felt the angina pain. But the doctor also advised Claude that the best way to avoid more radical treatment down the line was to exercise regularly and eat a low-fat diet.

Today, Claude carries nitroglycerin tablets with him wherever he goes and takes them only when he experiences the pain. He eats foods with low or no cholesterol or fat, and he continues to work in his garden as much as ever. He's even tilled up more of the backyard in order to make room for five more rows—his grandchildren want to plant pumpkins and watermelon to sell roadside for extra money.

BLACK MEN ARE AT GREATER RISK OF DEATH FROM HEART DISEASE

According to the American Heart Association, there were 953,110 deaths from cardiovascular disease in 1997.[2] Coronary heart disease death rates are higher among men than among women and are higher among blacks than among whites. In 1997, the death rate from cardiovascular disease was 438.2 per 100,000 for white males and 542.0 per 100,000 for black males.[3] The American Heart Association estimates that in 2000, cardio-vascular diseases and stroke cost $326.6 billion in direct and indirect costs.[4]

Though the heart disease death rate has been declining in recent years, it is declining more slowly among black men and

---

"The leading causes of death for African Americans in 1996 included ischemic heart disease, lung cancer, cerebrovascular disease, HIV/AIDS, unintentional injuries, prostate cancer, homicide, diabetic complications, breast cancer, pneumonia, influenza, chronic obstructive pulmonary disease, and perinatal conditions. **African Americans died from several of these diseases at dramatically greater rates than the overall population.** For example, in 1996 African Americans died at twice the rate from prostate cancer and diabetic complications than the overall population, and the age-adjusted mortality rate for stroke for the black population was two-thirds higher than that for the overall population."

Reprinted from Office of Minority Health, "Healthy People 2000: Progress Review for Black Americans," p. 8.

women than in the white population.[5] Because these declines in deaths related to heart disease are partly due to lifestyle changes, the differences between black and white men may be because white men have been assumed by both the media and the medical establishment to be at greatest risk. Thus, they have been more effectively targeted for prevention and treatment than have women and blacks. But the fact remains that black men are at even greater risk of heart-related deaths than white men.

HOW CAN I PREVENT HEART DISEASE?

Because making lifestyle changes can greatly reduce your risk of death from heart disease, it is important to know how you can make these changes a part of your life. What follows are simple prevention techniques you can use to prevent both heart disease and stroke—conditions that we discuss in the second part of this chapter:

- Stop smoking

- Fight obesity

- Lower bad cholesterol

- Avoid fast food

- Reduce your stress

For more information about all these prevention techniques, see Chapter 2.

CONTROL HIGH BLOOD PRESSURE

Another important way to prevent heart disease is to keep your blood pressure at a normal level. Hypertension (high blood pressure), which we discussed in depth in Chapter 3, is a major risk factor for heart disease and stroke. The prevalence of hypertension among black men ages 20 and older is nearly 1.5 times greater than among white men of the same age.[6]

Your chance of having a heart attack rises as your blood pressure rises. If you have high blood pressure, you have a three to four times greater risk of developing coronary heart disease than someone with normal blood pressure. According to the American Heart Association, compared with whites, blacks have a 1.3 times greater rate of nonfatal stroke, a 1.8 times greater rate of fatal stroke, a 1.5 times greater rate of heart disease death, and a 4.2 times greater rate of end stage kidney disease.[7] There are several strategies you can use to lower your blood pressure. See Chapter 3 for a more comprehensive discussion of these.

WHAT ABOUT UNAVOIDABLE RISKS?

Although there are major risk factors that you can reduce or eliminate from your life, others, such as socioeconomic class, heredity, age, and being male, are difficult or impossible to change. Blacks who have lower educational levels and who have low incomes are more likely to have higher blood pressure. Living in areas of instability and high social stress, as well as constantly grappling with educational and occupational insecurity, may increase your blood pressure, putting you at greater risk for heart disease and stroke. If you're in a low socioeconomic class, you may also not have access to quality medical care. Blacks make fewer visits to their doctors, and for many medical care is often inaccessible.

As we mentioned earlier, if heart disease runs in your family, you may have an increased risk of suffering from it. It's also important to remember that heart disease is diagnosed more often in people over age 50, so although you can't control your age, you *can* be sure to see a physician regularly. Even if some of your personal risk factors can't be changed, you do have control over many things, some of which we've mentioned already. It is in your power to decrease your likelihood of developing heart disease and increase your likelihood of living a long, healthy life.

HOW DO I KNOW IF I HAVE HEART DISEASE?

One way to tell if you have a particular illness or disease is to look for changes that you can see and feel. With heart disease, this search can be confusing because many times symptoms of other health disorders mimic those associated with heart disease. The primary indications of heart disease are:

- Rapid pounding of your heart

- Swelling in your legs

- Shortness of breath

- Pain located generally in the center of your chest

- Fainting

If you experience any of these, it doesn't automatically mean you have heart disease. Only by working with your physician or primary health care provider will you be able to determine exactly what caused the physical changes you're going through. But because heart disease is not something to be taken lightly, if you experience *any* of the sensations listed here, talk to a medical professional immediately. If you don't have a doctor, go to the emergency room. The better informed you are when you get there about the symptoms and the examination and treatment you may require, the better your chances are for good treatment.

MEDICAL DETECTION TECHNIQUES

There are many different ways your health care professional can determine if you have heart disease. The first—and least expensive—method is simply to listen to your heart. Your heart makes two sounds: "lubb" and "dubb." These sounds are made by the closing of the four valves we described earlier. If your doctor hears sounds other than these through the stethoscope, it may indicate that you have a heart problem.

If your doctor suspects heart trouble, there are many other tests he or she can order to make an accurate diagnosis. A few of the more common tests are:

- An *electrocardiogram (EKG or ECG)* records your heart's electrical activity to help your doctor detect any changes in the health of your heart. When giving you an EKG, the health provider will attach small wires to various areas of your body. These wires are connected to the electrocardio- gram machine, which will trace the patterns of electrical activity within your heart.

- *Chest x-rays* can show if your heart is enlarged or displaced within your chest cavity.

- Your doctor can also order a test called an *echocardio*gram, which generates sound waves that can detect motion of your heart and details of its valves and wall.

- Your doctor may also ask you to undergo a *cardiac catheterization,* a procedure in which dye is injected into your heart and its vessels. X-rays taken while the dye is in your body can portray your heart and its vessels in detail.

If, after the test results come back from one of these procedures, you are diagnosed with heart disease, it's essential that you make lifestyle changes and comply closely with the treatment plan your doctor prescribes. Otherwise, the consequences can be deadly.

MALCOLM'S STORY

The day of Malcolm's company picnic was glorious. The lake site had horseshoes, a pool, badminton, and volleyball for the employees and their families. From the volleyball court, Malcolm looked over at his wife and smiled. Then he noticed a slightly overweight man sitting at the picnic table next to her. The man's hand was resting over his chest, and his skin was very pale. More important, there was panic in the man's eyes. Malcolm had seen these very same signs in his own father when he was having a heart attack.

Malcolm ran toward the man, yelling over his shoulder to his surprised teammates to call an ambulance. But he knew that by the time the paramedics arrived it could be too late. Malcolm reached the man just as he was slumping off the picnic table bench and caught him just in time to keep his head from bumping on the concrete patio.

Malcolm then searched for the man's pulse: There wasn't one. He stretched the man out on the ground, tore open his shirt, loos-

ened his belt, and began CPR, which he had learned at the Red Cross. Malcolm continued to administer CPR until he heard sirens in the distance. By then, the color was coming back to the man's face. Malcolm stopped then and checked for a pulse. The man's pulse, although weak, had returned.

The paramedics arrived and transported the man to the hospital. It turned out the man, whose name was Larry, worked on the floor below Malcolm's office, so Malcolm could keep tabs on him. Larry survived the trip to the hospital and recovered nicely. Since his brush with death, Larry has changed his diet, lost some weight, and is exercising regularly. After that weekend, Malcolm's office sponsored a mandatory CPR class for all its employees.

SAVING LIVES WITH CPR

Sometimes, the heart completely stops beating or simply quivers, which means that although there is movement from the heart, it is not pumping blood. When the heart stops, cardiopulmonary resuscitation (CPR) can maintain blood flow to the heart and the rest of the body until medical therapy can begin.

If someone's heart stops beating, it is necessary to apply CPR to keep the heart pumping blood to the lungs and brain until medical help arrives to start the heart beating on its own again. Heart muscle tissue can die within five minutes after the heart stops beating. And it takes only four to six minutes for the brain to suffer irreversible damage. Serious or complete loss of brain function (sometimes called "brain death") can occur if the victim doesn't receive medical treatment within 10 minutes. You can never be sure when someone's heart may stop beating and CPR will be necessary. The more people who know CPR, the more lives can be saved.

Consider taking a CPR course, such as those offered by the American Red Cross, for hands-on experience—you could quite possibly save someone's life. Further, suggest to your employer or employees the possibility of having a CPR instructor come to your office to teach you and your co-workers this lifesaving skill.

TYPES OF HEART DISEASE

There are different causes and types of heart disease: Some people are born with heart defects (referred to as "congenital" heart defects). These congenital heart defects either appear at birth or develop over time, and may run in families. Doctors are currently studying how to diagnose and treat these disorders in children before they're even born. Other types of heart disease are caused by lifestyle factors, which we've already reviewed.

Atherosclerosis

Atherosclerosis (hardening of the arteries) occurs when the inner lining of your arteries is injured as a result of high blood pressure, elevated cholesterol, or toxins from smoke inhalation. Your arteries can be scarred, especially from smoking, and cholesterol deposits can cause your arteries to stiffen and the inner walls to narrow or clog. If your artery walls have narrowed, your blood may clot in its attempt to pass through the artery. This clotting can partially or completely obstruct the vessel, which can cause a heart attack or stroke.

When atherosclerosis blocks one of your coronary arteries (vessels located on the surface of and in your heart, which supply your heart with nourishment), part of your heart's blood supply can be cut off. That blockage can produce a symptom called angina or even a heart attack.

Angina

Angina, from the Greek root *anchoni,* means "strangulation." Angina is a sensation of heaviness or tightness in your chest, usually near or over your breastbone, sometimes radiating down the left arm and shoulder or spreading in fan fashion to your jaw. People feel angina pain in different ways. Some people describe it as a "full" feeling. But it is generally described as a frightening and oppressive feeling that can be accompanied by sweating, aching, and shortness of breath. Patients often experience it as is if someone were sitting on their chest.

Since angina attacks occur when your heart muscle doesn't receive as much blood as it needs, activities such as exercise, anxiety, or even eating, which require more blood flow, are most likely to bring on an attack. Angina can also occur while you're resting or sleeping, and may be a warning sign of an impending heart attack.

Heart Attack

When atherosclerosis (see Figure 4D) becomes so severe that it closes off one of your coronary arteries, you have a heart attack. Also called a "myocardial infarction," a heart attack sometimes produces symptoms that are similar to angina, but worse. The part of your heart that is served by the blocked artery is now cut off from its blood supply. Although damage to your heart muscle can begin in only a few minutes, with the use of a class of drugs called "clot busters" this damage can be reversed within the first six hours.

Pain or pressure are major symptoms of a heart attack, but the pain, though sometimes severe, can be so mild that you might dismiss it as indigestion or an aching muscle. Sometimes, there's

ATHEROSCLEROSIS

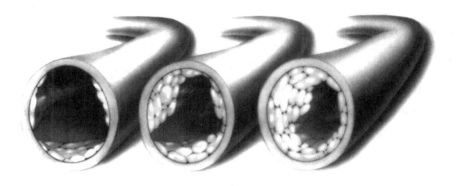

Reprinted with permission of the American Heart Association, "Heart and Stroke Facts" (1999), p. 4.

A CORONARY ARTERY THAT HAS BECOME NARROWED OR CLOGGED

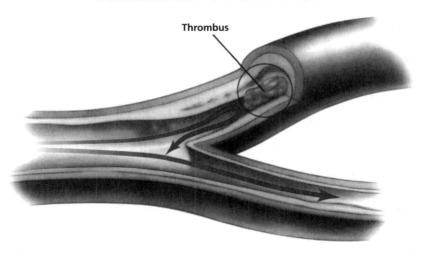

Reprinted with permission of the American Heart Association, "Heart and Stroke Facts" (1999), p. 38.

no pain at all, and you might simply complain of chest discomfort or tightness. The fact is that you don't have to experience pain or symptoms to suffer a heart attack. One out of every four heart attack victims experiences no symptoms at all. Such cases are called "silent" heart attacks. If you already suffer from angina when an attack occurs, you can tell the difference between angina and a heart attack by the fact that the pain of a heart attack will usually not lessen when you rest or take a nitroglycerin tablet.

People who have had massive heart attacks describe the experience as a very heavy, crushing feeling. The pain, they say, is usually centered under their breastbone. Some heart attack victims report pain in their back, between their shoulders, as well as in their left arm, jaw, shoulder, or neck. Heart attack victims may also sweat, be short of breath, or feel nauseated and vomit. It's essential to get medical help as quickly as possible if you think that you are having a heart attack or someone around you is: Don't wait around to see if the condition eases. Seek medical attention immediately because the heart may stop or beat so irregularly that the brain won't receive any blood for nourishment. While you're waiting for help, try to keep the person as calm as possible. If possible, get the victim to swallow two crushed aspirins with water—or without water if none is handy. If the heart has stopped, practice CPR!

Heart Failure

Heart failure occurs when your heart fails to perform adequately as a pump. This can result in the backup of fluid in your lungs and elsewhere in the body, causing shortness of breath or swelling in your legs or abdomen. Inadequate blood flow to the heart, heart attacks, infection, or inflammation (destruction caused by infection or other problems) can all cause an unhealthy heart muscle. Your heart can fail from prolonged high blood pressure, coronary artery disease, a viral illness, alcohol or other toxin overuse, or congenital heart disease.

Keep in mind that not all people who experience heart failure die from it—heart failure means only that the heart's pumping action is not adequate and needs to be treated.

Enlargement of the Heart

Just as weightlifting causes your muscles to become bigger and stronger, when your heart has to work harder to pump blood through your body (when you have hypertension, for example), the muscle builds and your heart becomes bigger. Unfortunately, in the case of the heart, bigger isn't better. Instead, the bigger your heart grows, the more difficult it is for it to work efficiently. If your heart is enlarged, it is probably weakened and less able to perform its functions. (To gain a better understanding of how to avoid or lessen the effects of high blood pressure, see Chapter 3.)

Arrhythmia

An arrhythmia is an abnormal heartbeat that occurs when there's any variation to the normal lubb-dubb rhythm of your heart. Sometimes an arrhythmia is dangerous because it can cause your heart to pump less efficiently. Such irregularities are often associated with dizziness, fainting, or chest pain. *Ventricular fibrillation*, the most serious type of rhythm disorder, can cause your ventricle to quiver and prevent your heart from pumping out any blood at all. When a patient has ventricular fibrillation, it may be necessary to "jump-start" the heart with an electric shock.

An artificial pacemaker is another possible treatment for arrhythmia. A pacemaker is a tiny device placed near your heart that can either stimulate your heart continuously or begin working only if your heart rate falls below a certain level.

Heart Valve Disorders

Your valves, or the doors located within your heart, are also potential danger zones. Congenital heart diseases (heart defects that appear at birth) and rheumatic heart disease can cause your valves to get stuck, and fail to open and close correctly. Doctors can surgically correct many congenital heart diseases.

Other heart valve disorders that at one time commonly resulted from strep infections, such as rheumatic fever, have been largely eliminated in the United States since the introduction of penicillin. However, these disorders are still common in underdeveloped countries where people have poor access to health care.

SECTION TWO: STROKE

Stroke is another form of cardiovascular disease, and occurs when your brain's blood supply is interrupted by a blocked blood vessel or when a blood vessel in your brain bursts, causing bleeding, also know as hemorrhage. When these things happen, your brain cells are deprived of oxygen and die.

According to the American Heart Association, young African Americans have a two to three times greater risk of ischemic stroke, and are 2.5 times more likely to die of a stroke than their white counterparts.[8] (Ischemic strokes are caused by an oxygen deficiency that can be caused by a constriction or obstruction in the blood vessel that supplies that part of the brain.) They also

AGE-ADJUSTED STROKE DEATH RATES

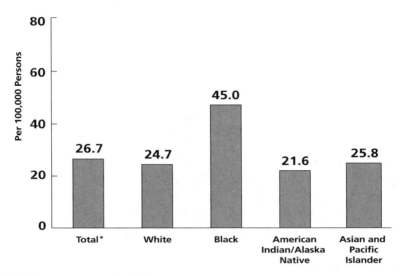

* All figures are age-adjusted

Reprinted from JNC VI.

report that when considered separately from other cardiovascular diseases, stroke ranks as the third leading cause of death in the United States; stroke claimed 159,791 lives in 1997,[9] and is also a leading cause of serious, long-term disability.[10] Approximately 600,000 people in the United States have a stroke every year.[11]

WHAT IS MY CHANCE OF HAVING A STROKE?

Your risk of having a stroke is greater if you are black, male, over 65 years of age, have diabetes, or if you or someone in your family has already had a stroke. Unfortunately, these are risk factors that you can't change. Other risk factors, as we've said, include lifestyle, diet, poor access to medical care, lack of awareness and research in the area of black men's health, and racial discrimination.

Furthermore, if you live in an area called the "Stroke Belt," a region that includes certain southeastern states, you're more likely to have a stroke. According to some experts, blacks in the Stroke Belt are 1.5 times more likely to suffer a stroke than whites.[13] One possible reason is that black people's diets within these areas tend to be high in cholesterol and saturated fats.

WARNING SIGNS OF A STROKE

There are many signs and symptoms of an impending stroke. The American Heart Association reports that you can possibly avert or lessen damage from a stroke by recognizing the following warning signals and seeking immediate medical attention:

- Sudden blurred or decreased vision in one or both eyes

- Numbness, weakness, and paralysis of the face, upper or lower limbs, on one or both sides of the body

- Difficulty speaking or understanding

- Dizziness, loss of balance, or unexplained falling

- Difficulty swallowing

- Headache (usually severe and of abrupt onset) or an unexplained change in the pattern of headaches

If you experience any of these symptoms, alone or in any combination, consult your doctor immediately.

TYPES OF STROKES

There are many different types of strokes.

Cerebral thrombosis is the most common type of stroke. Thrombotic strokes account for 60 percent of all strokes and generally occur in people over the age of 65. A thrombotic stroke occurs when an artery leading to your brain is blocked or clogged by a blood clot, or when the wall of one of your arteries thickens. (For more information about this, see the section on atherosclerosis earlier in this chapter.)

A cerebral embolism may occur when an artery leading to your brain is clogged by an embolus—a blood clot that has traveled from another area of your body.

Cerebral hemorrhages occur less frequently than the two stroke forms listed. A cerebral hemorrhage occurs when an artery in your brain bursts because of a weakening of its wall. All forms of brain hemorrhage can result in serious damage to the brain and even death. One cause of the weakening of the arterial wall is that a blood vessel hasn't formed normally as your brain develops. More commonly, the wall of the blood vessel becomes weak as the result of longstanding high blood pressure. You can help prevent this cause of brain hemorrhage by detecting and treating hypertension early.

All types of strokes can result in brain damage since the brain cannot repair itself when it is deprived of oxygen and other important forms of nourishment. The most important way to prevent brain damage is to prevent strokes in the first place. So, maintain a healthy lifestyle and treat abnormal conditions—such as hypertension and high blood fat levels—promptly.

TREATMENT FOR HEART DISEASE AND STROKE

Having heart disease or even a stroke doesn't mean your life is over. As Claude found out after his scare in the garden, the quality of your life depends on whether you're willing to take an active role in your health care. Monitor your blood pressure, control your blood cholesterol through diet, exercise, and eat a healthy diet to prevent heart disease from striking sometime in the future.

If you fall into one or more of the risk groups for heart disease or stroke, pay close attention to the preventive measures we've discussed here and in Chapter 2. Follow the advice of your doctor, health educator, or other health specialist. You'll increase your chances of preventing cardiovascular disease.

RESOURCES

American Heart Association
7272 Greenville Ave.
Dallas, TX 75231
(800) AHA-USA1 (800-242-8721) Customer Heart and Stroke Information
(888) 4-STROKE (888-478-7653) (Stroke Information)
http://www.americanheart.org
(The Association offers information, referrals, booklets, brochures, and community education programs.)

The Mended Hearts, Inc.
7272 Greenville Avenue
Dallas, Texas 75231-4596
(800) AHA-USA1 (800-242-8721) (Ask for Mended Hearts)
(214) 706-1442 (Home Office)
http://www.mendedhearts.org
(This is a support group for people who have gone through a heart attack, heart surgery, or angioplasty. Look up the chapter near you or write to the organization for more information.)

National Heart, Lung, and Blood Institute
NHLBI Information Center
P.O. Box 30105
Bethesda, MD 20824-0105
(301) 592-8573
http://www.nhlbi.nih.gov
Heart Health Toll-Free Information Line: 800-575-WELL (9355)
(The Center offers publications on heart disease, high blood pressure, and other topics.)

National Institute of Neurological Disorders and Stroke
Office of Communications and Public Liaison
P.O. Box 5801
Bethesda, MD 20824
(800) 352-9424
(301) 496-5751
(The Institute offers free brochures about strokes.)

National Rehabilitation Information Center
1010 Wayne Avenue
Suite 800
Silver Spring, MD 20910
(800) 346-2742 (Voice, U.S. only)
(301) 562-2400 (Voice)
(301) 495-5626 (TTY)
http://www.naric.com
(The Center provides some brochures, but mainly provides article reprints for a fee.)

National Stroke Association
96 Inverness Drive East
Suite I
Englewood, CO 80112-5311
(303) 649-9299
(800) STROKES (800-787-6537)
http://www.stroke.org
(This Association offers information on stroke support groups, videos, pamphlets, booklets, and brochures.)

NOTES FOR CHAPTER 4

1. American Heart Association "2000 Heart and Stroke Statistical Update." Source: http://www.americanheart.org/statistics/03cardio.html
2. Ibid.
3. Ibid.
4. American Heart Association, "Economic Cost of Cardiovascular Disease," 1999. Source: http://www.americanheart.org/statistics/10econom.html
5. U.S. Department of Health and Human Services. Healthy People 2010 (Conference Edition, in two volumes). Washington, DC: January 2000. For sale by the U.S. Government Printing Office, Superintendent of Documents, Washington, DC 20402-9382, Stock Number 017-001-

00543-6, ISBN 0-16-050260-8. For more information about Healthy People 2010 or to access Healthy People 2010 documents online, visit: http://www.health.gov/healthypeople/ or call 800-367-4725.

6. American Heart Association "2000 Heart and Stroke Statistical Update."
7. Ibid.
8. American Heart Association, "2000 Heart and Stroke Statistical Update." Source: http://www.americanheart.org/statistics/05stroke.html
9. African Americans and Cardiovascular Diseases Biostatistical Fact Sheets, American Heart Association, 1999. Source: http://www.americanheart.org/statistics/biostats/bioafr.htm
10. Ibid.
11. Ibid.
12. American Heart Association Press Release, NR 97-4530, May 13, 1997.
13. Ibid.

FIVE

Diabetes

JACK'S STORY: DIABETES UNDER CONTROL

"He was tall, big, and dashing, and I loved him so much," Deborah says, as she shares memories of Jack, her godfather. "I was a teenager when I heard he had diabetes, but at the time I didn't understand what diabetes was. I'd never heard him talk about it, and he never seemed sick to me."

DIABETES AND THE IMPORTANCE OF INSULIN

Unless you have diabetes, you probably can't explain what it is. After all, you can't see it. Most people know only that it has something to do with insulin and sugar. And many people still think that diabetes isn't serious. For people with the illness, though, diabetes is a lot more than just a "sugar problem."

Here's the story. The pancreas produces the hormone "insulin," which helps your body use glucose (sugar) for energy and general good health. (The pancreas sends the insulin into

103

your bloodstream when it's needed.) As the amount of sugar in your blood rises, your pancreas detects the increase and sends out a "message" into your bloodstream via insulin. This insulin "message" causes all of your cells to take the sugar out of your blood and use it for energy. When your blood sugar level is low, your pancreas doesn't send the insulin, so your body holds onto the little sugar you have instead of using it for energy. (You always have some sugar in your bloodstream because your brain can't function without it.)

When you develop diabetes all this changes. Either your pancreas becomes unable to produce insulin or your cells are unable to receive the insulin "message." As a result, your body can no longer efficiently use the food you eat or control the amount of sugar in your bloodstream.

DIABETES AND BLACKS

More than 15 million people—that's almost 6 percent of the U.S. population—have diabetes. For blacks the disease is even more prevalent: About 2.3 million (or 10.8 percent) of all African Americans have diabetes. This means that we're nearly twice as likely to suffer from it.

Here's the scariest statistic of all: One-third of us don't know we have it!

For seniors, the illness is even more widespread because 25 percent of blacks between the ages of 65 and 74 have the disease.[1] Each day, roughly 2,200 people are diagnosed with diabetes; about 798,000 people will be diagnosed this year.[2] And although researchers have found many ways to control and prevent diabetes, there's still no cure.

People with diabetes are at increased risk of developing additional medical complications such as blindness, kidney disease, amputations, heart attack, and stroke. These complications make diabetes the seventh leading cause of death in the United States.[3] Several studies report that diabetes-related complications are more frequent among blacks. In 1999, diabetic nephropathy (kidney damage from diabetes) accounted for 39 percent of the cases of end stage renal disease (ESRD) among black patients in the United States.[4] Diabetic ESRD is three to six times more common in blacks than in whites.[5]

WHAT CAUSES DIABETES AND HOW CAN I PREVENT IT?

Though certain people have a greater tendency to get diabetes than others, no one knows exactly what causes the disease. Certainly, heredity is a factor, as are rapid weight gain, inflammation of the pancreas, or other illnesses.

Keeping your weight at a healthy level and avoiding "quick cure" diets may help to prevent the disease. (Eight out of ten people who are diagnosed with adult onset diabetes are overweight.) Obesity is a major cause of diabetes; more than 80 percent of all people with type 2 diabetes are obese. The problem here is that insulin doesn't work properly if you're overweight. Here's why: On the outside of each of your cells are areas called insulin receptor sites. As the name suggests, these sites are where insulin attaches itself to the cell and where blood glucose enters. If you're obese, these insulin receptor sites are less effective because your body's ability to transport glucose into the cell is diminished. Therefore, your body may become resistant to insulin.

(Following the guidelines for general good health outlined in Chapter 2 may help you to prevent or delay the onset of the disease.)

TYPES OF DIABETES

There are two main types of diabetes: type 1 and type 2. There are a few secondary types of diabetes, as well.

TYPE 1 DIABETES

Type 1 diabetes, formerly known as "insulin-dependent diabetes," usually occurs in children and young adults, although it can strike at any age. Approximately 1 million people in the United States have this type of diabetes.

If you suffer from type 1 diabetes, you have little or no insulin in your body and must take daily insulin injections to survive. When insulin isn't available, the cells in your body can starve because sugar isn't allowed to pass into the cells. At the same time, your liver produces excess amounts of glucose, which remains useless in your blood.

HOW DO I KNOW IF I HAVE TYPE 1 DIABETES?

According to the American Diabetes Association, the common symptoms of type 1 diabetes are:

- Frequent urination (and/or bed-wetting in children)

- Losing weight without trying

- Extreme hunger

- Extreme thirst

- Extreme weight loss

- Weakness and fatigue

- Feeling edgy and moody

- Feeling sick to your stomach and vomiting

- Blurred vision

- Going into a coma

If you experience any of these symptoms, see your doctor immediately.

TYPE 2 DIABETES

Type 2, formerly known as "noninsulin-dependent diabetes," the more common type of the disease, accounts for 90 percent of the cases. Type 2 diabetes usually occurs in overweight adults older than age 40, which is why it's sometimes referred to as "adult onset diabetes." Recently, there has been an increase in type 2 diabetes diagnosed in children. These children tend to have the same risk factors (obesity, sedentary lifestyle) as adults. The majority of blacks who have diabetes have type 2 diabetes.

Type 2 diabetes occurs when your pancreas doesn't make enough insulin or when your body can't adequately use the insulin your pancreas does produce. If you have type 2 diabetes, you may be able to manage your condition by eating a healthy diet. But eating well isn't your only key to managing the disease: The fact is, both the quality and length of your life will depend primarily on how committed you are to being an active participant in your own health care. By taking control, many people with type 2 diabetes have lived full, happy, healthy lives, often living longer than their friends who don't have the disease. By following the diet and lifestyle guidelines recommended to keep your disorder in check, you'll help to control your diabetes and improve your overall health, too.

HOW DO I KNOW IF I HAVE TYPE 2 DIABETES?

Type 2 diabetes tends to run in some families; in fact, several members of each generation may develop the disease. If your family has a history of diabetes, you should be tested periodically, especially after you reach age 40, or if you're overweight. The symptoms of type 2 diabetes, unlike those of type 1, are sometimes so mild that you might not even know that you're sick. If you think you may be at risk, look for these signs and symptoms:

- Fatigue

- Frequent urination, especially at night

- Unusual thirst

- Sudden weight loss

- Blurred vision or any vision changes

- Slow healing of skin, gums, and urinary tract infections

- Tingling or numbness in feet, legs, or fingers

- Frequent skin infections

- Irritability

If you detect any of these symptoms, see your doctor immediately.

Sometimes, however, you can have diabetes without being aware of any symptoms at all. For instance, though you may not notice any symptoms, you may have a medical history of glucose (sugar) in your urine or a gradual increase in your blood glucose level over several months or years. In older people, a doctor may discover diabetes during a routine physical exam, or when a person is hospitalized for another reason. People may not notice any symptoms, which is why it's so important to be tested for diabetes regularly.

HOW TO CONTROL DIABETES

Although diabetes is serious, it's not a death sentence. Your health depends on how you choose to manage your condition. Remember: *You're in control.* You can sit back and let the disease run its course—and ruin your life—or you can pay close attention to what your body needs and take care of those needs.

In truth, the "diabetic lifestyle" is one that everyone should adopt! For a diabetic, what's essential is what should be essential for all of us: eat well, exercise regularly, and pay close attention to the signs and signals of your body. Having diabetes can be a great excuse to get your whole family involved in living a healthy lifestyle.

People with diabetes are part of a health care team—one that includes your physician, health educator, nutritionist, eye doctor, foot doctor, and others who specialize in common complications of diabetes. There will be times when you need the help of all your teammates, but you're still the team captain. To know when to seek help, you need to understand your condition. *You're the one who needs to monitor your body day in and day out to* become aware of the warning signs that tell you that it's time to rely on another team member.

MONITORING YOUR CONDITION

To monitor your health effectively, start making routine visits to your doctor three or four times a year. (If you develop additional health problems, you may need to visit your doctor more often.) The doctor will usually check your weight, blood pressure, and pulse; listen to your heart at every visit; and examine your eyes and feet. (We'll explain why later in this chapter.)

In addition, periodically your doctor will monitor your glucose control with a blood test for "glycosylated hemoglobin," also called hemoglobin A_1 or hemoglobin A_{1c}. This test gives you and your doctor information about your average blood glucose control for the eight-week period preceding the test. Hemoglobin A_{1c} levels correlate with your risk for developing complications.

One of your jobs as team captain will be to monitor your blood glucose two or three times a week, or perhaps more often if you're taking insulin. Your health care professional (doctor, nurse, or diabetes educator) will tell you how often you need to test your blood sugar. You should have an established schedule geared to your individual needs.

HOW DO I TEST MY BLOOD SUGAR?

Many products are available that test your blood glucose levels, such as lancets, which you use to prick your finger to get a small drop of blood; test strips, which you read by comparing the color on the strip to a color chart; and blood glucose monitors, which automatically read test strips and show your exact blood glucose level. Your health care professional can help you determine the method that is best for you and instruct you how to use it.

Keep records of the numbers you've recorded—one for yourself and one for your doctor to see at your next checkup. Your doctor can use the information to identify problems and to correct them by making changes to your insulin dose, your diet, or your exercise program.

Once a year, you should get a thorough physical examination, during which your doctor should pay special attention to your cholesterol and triglyceride levels. Ideally, your cholesterol level should be below 200 milligrams and your triglyceride level below 150 milligrams. You can also have an EKG (electrocardiogram) and other diagnostic tests done to evaluate your risk of any long-term complications.

During this examination, your doctor will also do urine and blood tests to check your kidneys. In addition, he or she should do an in-depth evaluation of your blood pressure by taking it several times. If your blood pressure is above 130/85, you may be put on a program to reduce it to a lower, more "normal" blood pressure level.

You should also have your eyes thoroughly examined once a year by an eye doctor (ophthalmologist). This is very important because treatments are available that can help prevent blindness, a common complication of diabetes.

HOW DO I KNOW IF I NEED INSULIN INJECTIONS?

If you have type 1 diabetes, you're insulin-dependent, which means you'll need daily insulin injections. (Some people with type 2 diabetes also need to take insulin.) If you're on insulin therapy, your doctor will develop a custom-made plan that best suits your needs. After checking your blood sugar, you and your doctor will be able to tell how much insulin you'll need throughout each day.

JACK TAKES DIABETES IN STRIDE

When Deborah saw her godfather again, she asked him about his diabetes. Jack said he'd had it since he was a teenager. "It's nothing for you to worry about. It takes me less time to take care of my condition than it takes you to put on your makeup," he assured her. Indeed, Deborah couldn't remember seeing her godfather slowed down by his condition. In fact, Jack was probably the most energetic, happy-go-lucky man she had ever met!

This conversation made Deborah curious about her godfather's diabetes, so she asked him to show her how he treated it. He was delighted with her interest. "Tell you what," he said, "I'm due for my afternoon injection. C'mon, and I'll show you how I do it."

He showed her the insulin supply he kept in the refrigerator and the individually wrapped syringes stored in the medicine cabinet. Then Jack pulled up his shirt and scrubbed an area on his abdomen with soap and water. Deborah, wary of needles, flinched when he pushed the needle into his abdomen, but Jack remarked, "I've been doing this for years. It's like brushing my teeth."

HOW DO I TAKE THE INJECTIONS?

Your doctor or nurse will show you how best to take insulin injections. But just to give you an idea, we'll give you some pointers, too. You'll need to inject your insulin into the fatty tissue under your skin, instead of into a vein. That allows for better, more even absorption of the insulin into your bloodstream. Make sure you clean the top of the bottle of insulin and the site of the injection with rubbing alcohol, or soap and water.

You'll want to choose a different area of your body each time you give yourself an injection because if you use the same site each time, your skin can get irritated. Most people prefer to inject themselves in the abdomen, because insulin tends to be absorbed more slowly there than from areas such as your arm, leg, or hip. When your body absorbs insulin quickly, the effects don't last as long.

To take an insulin injection, follow these simple steps:

1. Pull back on the plunger of the needle to the number of units of insulin that you need.

2. Push the needle into the bottle and depress the plunger, which pushes air into the bottle.

3. Turn the insulin bottle upside down and draw the required amount of insulin into the syringe.

4. Tap the syringe, still inside the bottle, which will send the air bubbles to the top.

5. Push the plunger in slightly, which will force the air bubbles out of the syringe into the bottle.

6. Remove the syringe and check to make sure you've withdrawn the correct amount of insulin.

7. Pinch and pull up your skin at the injection site you've chosen, making sure it's fatty tissue, not muscle.

8. Take the syringe, push the needle straight into your skin, and depress the plunger slowly and evenly.

9. Dispose of the needle properly.

Researchers are always looking for ways to make managing your diabetes easier. Here are a few recent developments that make it still easier to give yourself an insulin injection:

- *Jet injectors* are needle-free and pressurized to deliver insulin directly into your bloodstream.

- *Insulin pens* look like fountain pens and contain insulin. With these pens, you don't need to carry around syringes and vials.

- *Insulin pumps* are in place all day and night. They slowly release insulin through a plastic tube, which is inserted through your skin.

Researchers are currently exploring ways to deliver insulin to your bloodstream by *inhaling the hormone*. What's more, *pancreas transplantation* may someday replace insulin injection for some patients. (Pancreas transplantation is when doctors replace the faulty insulin-producing cells in your pancreas with new ones that come from a human donor.)

CONTROL YOUR DIABETES THROUGH DIET

It's always a good idea to eat right—whether you have diabetes or not. So, if you have the disease, look at it as an opportunity to improve your overall health and control your diabetes. And enlist the help of your family and friends! Their support will make it easier for you to make the changes that you need to live a longer, healthier life. At the same time, they'll learn health tricks that might make their lives stronger, too.

Because people with diabetes commonly suffer from heart disease and high blood pressure, your nutrition plan must take all three of these conditions into account. Your diet should be high in complex carbohydrates such as breads, beans, pasta, potatoes, fruits, and other vegetables. These foods tend to raise your energy level for a longer period of time than will simple carbohydrates like the sugars in candy and cake. (Your body has a hard time producing enough insulin to burn sweets.)

Though fruit is loaded with lots of vitamins and minerals, you need to be careful with it. Natural sugar, or fructose, which is found in fruit, can increase your blood sugar level. If you have diabetes, it's okay for you to eat fruit and drink fruit juices, but limit your intake to the amounts that your dietitian or diabetes educator recommends. Always be aware of how much is too much: It can be a matter of life or death.

You should also limit your fat and cholesterol intake. Fat and cholesterol can attach to the inside walls of your arteries, making it hard for your blood to circulate. This hampered circulation can cause less blood to flow to your vital organs. Lack of blood flow can cause heart disease, kidney failure, or stroke. In extreme cases, bad circulation can make it necessary that toes, feet, or legs be amputated. Since people with diabetes are already at a high risk for these problems, lessen your chances of these complications by decreasing your intake of fat and cholesterol. (For more information on cholesterol, refer to Chapters 2 and 4 in this book.)

Here are a few ways to cut the fat:

- Limit meat portion sizes. Try to limit yourself to six ounces of meat per day, and get your proteins from other sources as often as possible.

- Use lean meats, such as fish and poultry. Choose meats that contain less than 3 grams of fat per ounce.

- Avoid high-fat meats, such as sausage, frankfurters, prime cuts of meats, luncheon meats, and organ meats (such as chitlins and liver).

- Cook to get rid of as much fat as possible. Broil, bake, and boil foods instead of frying them, and remove fat from meats before making gravies and sauces.

- Use skim milk. If you now drink whole milk, gradually change from 2 percent to 1 percent, then to skim.

- Use a margarine with liquid vegetable oil listed as the first ingredient. Tub margarine contains more unsaturated fat than stick margarine. (See Chapter 2 for a more detailed comparison of saturated and unsaturated fats.)

- Use liquid vegetable oils in place of solid whenever possible. Olive or canola oils are better for you than either butter or margarine.

- Limit your intake of eggs to three per week at the most. Eat egg whites instead of egg yolks.

- Use low-fat or no-fat dairy products. Substitute low-fat or no-fat yogurt for cream and mayonnaise. Select cheeses with fewer than 5 grams of fat per ounce.

- Whenever you can, try to find a low-fat or fat-free version of the foods you like to eat. Thousands of modified-fat products are available in grocery stores.

If you have diabetes, remember that what and how much you eat can be a matter of life or death. Besides cutting down the amount of fat you eat, you also need to cut back on salt because high levels of salt increase your risk of developing high blood pressure. People with diabetes are at higher risk of developing high blood pressure anyway, so why chance it? (See Chapter 3 for more information about hypertension.)

DEVELOP YOUR PERSONAL MEAL PLAN

Fast food isn't good for anyone since it's usually high in calories, sugar, salt, and cholesterol. But for a person with diabetes, eating these foods can be especially hazardous. Mealtime doesn't have to be a burden, though—you just need to remember that the ideal diet for a person with diabetes is the ideal diet for everyone. So plan your meals! Look at having diabetes as a reason to live a healthier lifestyle. A registered dietitian will help you come up with a flexible and enjoyable meal plan that's right for you. Although at first you may feel that your choices are limited, you'll soon find that there are plenty of foods out there that you can safely eat.

Because your diet is adjusted to your insulin intake—which should remain relatively stable—try to stay on a regular eating schedule. Never skip a meal if you take insulin, or you could upset the insulin–sugar balance. If you can't eat lunch at your

regular time, eat a snack to keep you going until you can eat a full
meal. A snack will help to prevent your blood glucose from drop-
ping too low. A good balance between your diet and insulin will
mean that your body is processing your food at the same time the
insulin in your body is peaking, or working hardest.

Changing your eating habits is one of the hardest lessons to
learn. This is especially true for black men because many tradi-
tionally African American foods are high in fat and salt. When we
work to change our eating habits, we're combating hundreds of

---

Your first job in controlling diabetes is sticking to a diet. In fact,
some people with type 2 diabetes can control their blood sugar simply by proper meal planning. Many people who develop type 2 diabetes are overweight or obese. ("Overweight" is defined as having a
body mass index of 25-29.9, while "obesity" is a BMI of 30 or
greater. BMI is simply one's weight in kilograms divided by height in
meters squared.)

BMI of 27 or greater is considered one of the risk factors
that will require screening for diabetes, even if the individual is
without symptoms. To put this another way, BMI of 27 or greater is
"a pre-diabetic state," especially is there is a family history of diabetes.

If you are overweight, the simplest and most cost-effective way
to reduce your risk of developing diabetes, or of managing the disease if you have it, is to lose weight. Your doctor or dietician can
help you plan a diet that's right for you. You'll be glad to learn that
what you eat can be tasty, even if it's healthy.

---

years of history and tradition. Keep in mind that because you've learned your eating habits over a lifetime, you won't be able to change them in a day, a week, or a month. Be patient with yourself and make changes gradually.

Because you need to become aware of your eating habits before you can change them, keep track of everything you eat and drink, how long it takes to eat your meals and snacks, where you eat, with whom you eat, what else you were doing while you were eating, and how hungry you were. If you keep accurate records, you'll notice that certain patterns start to appear. You'll be able to see, for example, just how many times you went to that fast-food restaurant because you were in a hurry. Or how many times you drank a glass of wine or a can of beer just to be sociable.

As you become more accustomed to your new way of eating, you need to be prepared to avoid situations where your eating problems occur. Be on the lookout for snack substitutes, such as low-fat crackers (with less than 2 grams of fat per serving), raw vegetables, and fresh fruit. And try to avoid walking past your favorite neighborhood candy store, even if it takes a little longer for you to get home. The exercise will make you feel better.

If you can't avoid certain food-tempting situations, implement a plan to eliminate problems and "limit the damage." If you do your own grocery shopping, make a shopping list and stick to it, and don't go with an empty stomach! Meal planning may take a little more time and effort, but the benefits will be worth it.

When you go to parties or restaurants, think ahead about what you're going to eat or order. (Here's a hint: If you order your meal first, you'll be less tempted by the foods other people are ordering.) Try to leave a little food on your plate at the end of each meal, and don't let anyone persuade you to "just take one more little bite." If you're sincere in your efforts to control your eating habits, you'll succeed. And you may notice that over time, other people will start to adopt your healthy eating habits, too!

JACK EXERCISES REGULARLY

Deborah noticed that her godfather, unlike a lot of other elderly people, didn't look overweight. In fact, even though Jack was 62, he was in great shape and kept his weight under control by exercising regularly. He either walked or rode his bike for 30 minutes every day— it was a rule he lived by. If it rained, he rode his stationary bicycle in the house, and during the winter, he walked in one of the local malls. He told Deborah that if it weren't for his daily exercise, he wouldn't feel nearly as good as he did. Deborah hadn't realized that Jack's exercise was a major part of his diabetes treatment.

THE BENEFITS OF REGULAR EXERCISE

Though everyone can benefit from regular exercise, it's especially good for you if you have diabetes. Why? Because food increases your blood sugar level, but exercise decreases it by increasing your body's sensitivity to insulin. Aerobic exercise, such as walking, jogging, biking, or swimming, is the best exercise for general fitness and for controlling your blood glucose.

WHAT COMPLICATIONS CAN I DEVELOP
IF I HAVE DIABETES?

Black people are more likely than others to suffer from three serious diabetes complications: blindness, end stage renal disease (also known as ESRD or kidney failure), and amputations.[6] The longer your diabetes remains out of control, the more likely it is that you'll develop one or more of the following complications:

- *Your risk of developing heart disease and stroke increases*
  If you have diabetes, your risk of suffering from heart disease or stroke is two to four times higher because it's more likely that fat and cholesterol will cling to the walls of your blood vessels: When the blood vessels that nourish your heart become clogged, you can have a heart attack. And if the arteries leading to your brain become blocked, you can suffer a stroke because the blockage keeps your brain from receiving oxygen and nutrients. (For more information about heart disease and stroke, see Chapter 4.)

- *You can lose your sight*
  In people ages 20 to 74, diabetes is the leading cause of new cases of blindness. In fact, each year, diabetes causes 12,000 to 24,000 people to lose their sight, and blacks are twice as likely as whites to suffer from diabetes-related blindness.[7] If you've had diabetes for 15 years or longer, you're likely to develop some sort of damage to the blood vessels in your eye. Mild blood-vessel changes are called background retinopathy.

If you have diabetes, you may also have cataracts or glaucoma. All these problems can affect your vision and may lead to blindness. Usually the early stages of eye disease have no symptoms, which is why an annual visit to your eye doctor is extremely important, so that you can be treated before it's too late.

- *You're at a greater risk of developing kidney disease*
  Black people with diabetes are 2.6 to 5.6 times more likely to suffer from kidney disease than whites; in fact, doctors diagnose more than 4,000 new cases of end stage renal disease (ESRD) each year.[8]

  If your small blood vessels are damaged, it can affect your kidneys—a condition called *diabetic nephropathy.* Your doctor can tell if you have diabetic kidney disease by checking for excess protein in your urine, which indicates kidney damage. You may notice other signs, too: When you lose too much protein through your urine, your ankles swell and fluids can build up in your lungs. If you have advanced diabetic kidney disease, you probably also have high blood pressure, but if you can control it, you may be able to prevent or better manage diabetic kidney disease. (See Chapter 8 for more information about kidney disease.)

- *You may experience nerve damage*
  Neuropathy, or nerve damage, is the least understood of all the small blood vessel complications of diabetes. When the small blood vessels around your nerves become damaged by high blood glucose levels, your nerves aren't able to

function properly, which dulls the sensitivity of your nerve endings. Though diabetic neuropathy can affect any nerve in your body, it's most common in the feet and lower legs.

When neuropathy leads to a loss of sensation in your feet, you could suffer from an injury, infection, or burns from very hot water and not even realize it. Here's what happens: If the nerves in your feet are severely damaged, you can develop gangrene, which can spread throughout your feet and legs, requiring amputation. And among those people with diabetes, blacks are 1.5 to 2.5 times more likely to suffer from lower limb amputations.[9]

So if you have diabetes, make it part of your daily routine to check your feet and legs for possible cuts or infections, and see your doctor right away if you notice anything suspicious.

- *You can become impotent*
Another major complication of diabetes is impotence, which develops slowly over many months or years. Your erections become softer and less frequent until you can no longer get one at all. There are many new ways to treat impotence, though, so if your erections are changing, it's a good idea to talk to your doctor to find out which treatments would be best for you.

- *Your risk of developing skin and teeth problems increases*
People with diabetes are more prone to problems with their skin and teeth (such as periodontal disease) than others. In fact, gum disease is the main reason people lose their teeth

when they get older. Ask your dentist to show you how to prevent periodontal disease.

- *You may come up against hypoglycemia*
Hypoglycemia refers to low blood sugar (it's sometimes called an insulin reaction). Your blood sugar levels may drop if you're very physically active, if you've gone without a meal, or if you've taken too much insulin. Hypoglycemic symptoms can include trembling, sweating, hunger, and a rapid heartbeat. If you have diabetes and experience these symptoms, it could be an emergency; you need to replace your body's sugar by eating either a glucose tablet or a hard candy. (It's a good idea to keep glucose tablets or hard candies with you all the time in case you, or someone you know, should have an insulin reaction.)

THE GOOD NEWS

The good news is that you can delay or avoid the majority of these complications by keeping tight control over your blood sugar. A landmark study, the Diabetes Complications and Control Trial (DCCT), demonstrated that diabetic complications can be reduced up to 60 percent in patients with type 1 diabetes. The recently conducted United Kingdom Prospective Diabetes Study (UKPDS) also showed that tight blood glucose control can significantly reduce complications in people with type 2 diabetes. These two studies prove the importance of following the guidelines that we've outlined in this chapter to prevent diabetes-related complications from happening to you.

CONCLUSION

Now that you know the facts, it's up to you to determine how your diabetes will affect your life. It takes only about 10 minutes each day to control your diabetes, and most people can do it in even less time than that!

Remember that you're part of a well-educated team of health care providers. Your teammates can help you approach each aspect of your disease and tackle any challenges that may come up. Get a complete physical, check your blood sugar level regularly, plan your meals, watch your weight, and exercise regularly. By following these simple guidelines, like many other people with diabetes, you can grow old gracefully, too!

RESOURCES

American Association of Diabetes Educators
100 West Monroe Street
Fourth Floor
Chicago, IL 60603-1901
(312) 424-2426
http://www.aadenet.org/
(This is an organization of health professionals who provide diabetes education for patients. Visit their website to find a diabetes educator in your area.)

American Diabetes Association
1701 North Beauregard Street
Alexandria, VA 22311
(800) DIABETES (800-342-2383)
http://www.diabetes.org
(The Association gives information and referrals, and has quarterly journals and a newsletter. Their website contains a wealth of diabetes information.)

Juvenile Diabetes Foundation International
120 Wall Street
New York, NY 10005
(800) JDF-CURE (800-533-2873)
(212) 785-9500
(212) 785-9595 (fax)
http://www.jdf.org/
(Offers patient information about juvenile diabetes.)

National Diabetes Information Clearinghouse
1 Information Way
Bethesda, MD 20892-3560
(301) 654-3327
(301) 907-8906 (fax)
http://www.niddk.nih.gov/health/diabetes/ndic.htm
(The Clearinghouse offers brochures and fact sheets, newsletters, and an online database.)

NOTES FOR CHAPTER 5

1. American Diabetes Association, "Diabetes Facts and Figures," 1999.
2. Ibid.
3. Ibid.
4. Incidence and prevalence of ESRD. *USRDS Annual Report 1999*, pp. S40–62.
5. Carter, J. S., Pugh, J. A., Monterrosa, A., "Non-Insulin-Dependent Diabetes Mellitus in Minorities in the United States," *Annals of Internal Medicine*, 1996, vol. 125, pp. 221–232.
6. American Diabetes Association, "Diabetes Facts and Figures," 1999.
7. Ibid.
8. Ibid.
9. Ibid.

SIX

Cancer

LONNIE'S STORY

Lonnie, a novelist, was a man everyone envied. He was happily married, had six children, and appeared to be living a perfect life. His career, too, flourished. He'd written a dozen books, and nearly all of them had done well and were still in print.

But the constant threat of deadlines had made Lonnie's life increasingly stressful. He started smoking more often: it calmed him down, he said. Further, because of all the social functions he attended as a successful novelist, he began drinking more alcohol.

One winter, Lonnie developed a nagging cough, which he at first simply attributed to a winter cold. When it lingered, he blamed it on allergies. Finally, after several months, he went to a doctor to have it checked; that's when a chest x-ray revealed a small, isolated white spot the size of a quarter in Lonnie's lungs. He had cancer.

Most of us have known someone with cancer, and when we hear the word, we're immediately fearful, perhaps because cancer is

129

commonly misperceived as a death sentence. Many people don't realize that 50 percent of all cancer patients have more than a five-year survival rate, and many are cured!

So what is cancer? What determines who is cured and who isn't? How can you prevent it from happening to you?

WHAT CAUSES CANCER?

There are many different risk factors for developing cancer, the most common of which is aging itself. Everyone's risk of cancer is increasing because, as a population, we're living longer. And although many people diagnosed with cancer likely have no idea what caused it, the disease may be caused by an accumulation of different factors over a lifetime.

The greatest risk for cancer is old age. Therefore, taking preventive measures when you are young obviously offers enormous benefits. We discussed prevention in Chapter 2, but there are also specific preventive measures you can take to reduce your risk of cancer. Eating a high-fiber diet that's loaded with fruits and vegetables may have a strong protective effect against many cancers by limiting the amount of time that carcinogens—cancer-causing chemicals—remain in your body. (But a recent study has raised questions about this.) We can also help ourselves by avoiding alcohol and nicotine. Drinking alcohol and smoking both contribute to the formation of many common cancers, including cancers of the esophagus, larynx, mouth, and throat.

It's interesting to note that Seventh Day Adventists, a religious group, espouse a strictly vegetarian diet that contains great amounts of fruit, vegetables, and whole grains. They also avoid smoking, and drinking alcohol, tea, and coffee. As a population, they have been recorded to have one-half the rate of cancer of the general population![1]

Another cause of cancer is exposure to carcinogens. Although you may not think you're at risk, carcinogens often work silently, altering a cell's genetic code without your even knowing it. Once cells are altered and become cancerous, they may reproduce much more rapidly than normal cells or grow steadily without control. This out-of-control growth may allow cancerous cells to spread to other parts of your body.

Smoke contains carcinogens that increase your risk of lung, bladder, tongue, and larynx cancers, among others. If you smoke, quit—it's the most effective way to prevent many forms of cancer. Unfortunately, it's not so easy to recognize and avoid other carcinogens. Asbestos is a good example: For many years, asbestos was used in many work environments. But it was only when employees began to be diagnosed with cancer that asbestos was identified as a carcinogen.

Several government agencies, including the Occupational Safety and Health Administration (OSHA) and the National Institute of Occupational Safety (NIOS), now protect us from carcinogens in the workplace. The Food and Drug Administration (FDA) identifies carcinogens in drug and food additives, and the Environmental Protection Agency (EPA) attempts to control carcinogens in our air and water.

But despite that protection, and regardless of how careful you are about avoiding carcinogens, everyone is at risk, and that risk may be greater if someone in your family has had cancer. For Lonnie, as with many cancer patients, a number of factors probably contributed to his disease. For example, poor diet (you'll recall that Lonnie often ate party food) accounts for approximately 35 percent of cancer deaths. In Lonnie's case, and the case of many others, high stress levels may have compromised the immune system (Lonnie's resistance to disease). His social drinking could have changed the balance in his cells, making him more vulnerable to cancer. And of course, Lonnie's cigarette smoking probably played a major role: Cigarette smoke alone contains 40 known carcinogens, and almost half of all smokers between ages 35 and 69 suffer untimely deaths.

Whether you're fighting cancer or simply working for prevention, it's important to strive for balance and health in all areas of your life. (See Chapter 2 for more information about making lifestyle changes.)

WHY ARE BLACKS MORE LIKELY TO DIE OF CANCER THAN WHITES?

So now we've established some of the causes of cancer. But that doesn't explain the increased risk of cancer-related deaths in black Americans. Blacks have a higher adjusted cancer death rate than whites: Between 1990 and 1996, 308.8 out of 100,000 black males and 208.8 out of 100,000 white males died from cancer. For black females, the rate was 168.1 per 100,000 versus 139.8 per 100,000 for white females.[2]

There are many potential causes for these inequalities. Although some hereditary cancers seem to be more common among blacks, most cancers, such as lung cancer, are the direct result of environmental and lifestyle factors, as well as of lack of access to good health care. By learning how to take better care of ourselves, we may be able to reverse some of the statistics.

We don't pretend that that reversal will be easy. Many cancers are more often diagnosed in a localized stage—that is, before they've spread—among whites than among blacks. This means that by the time a black man's cancer has been diagnosed by a doctor, it may already have spread too much to be treated effectively. Early detection and timely treatment can increase your chance of survival.

But many blacks are at a distinct disadvantage. They may develop cancers early because of poverty, lack of access to medical care, and discrimination. Clearly, if we were able to make environmental and social changes *as well as* increase our own knowledge and awareness of medical and preventive strategies, cancer death rates would radically decrease among black men.

Here's another problem that bears on cancer and race. There are indications that if a person believes he or she can get well, his or her chance of being cured may increase. But national surveys indicate that blacks overestimate the deadliness of cancer and the prevalence of cancer prevalence in their population. Additionally, blacks are less knowledgeable about cancer warning signs and screening methods than are whites. So it appears that what is needed to improve the cancer picture among our people is not only early screening but also better information since, in this case, information has both practical and psychological benefits.

But what can we do about these differences between the awareness and outlook of blacks and white—differences that seem to account for the longer delay in seeking diagnosis and treatment among blacks and the greater occurrence among us of more advanced stages of cancer?

Because cancer may be partially avoidable with proper diet, a healthy lifestyle, and by reducing a variety of environmental risks, there are two steps that can help eradicate these racial discrepancies, and both of them involve education. First, *prevention* is the only cure with a 100 percent guarantee. Second, *early detec-*

tion can greatly increase your chances of surviving a cancer. By getting frequent checkups and specifically requesting diagnostic tests for cancer, you can help your doctor determine if you have cancer or if you're at risk. You can also detect cancer on your own by making it a habit to check your body for abnormalities frequently. If you notice any change in your energy level or if you see or feel spots, lumps, or physical symptoms that seem suspicious, ask your doctor about them. Later in this chapter, we will discuss common signs of cancer you should watch for.

LONNIE IS DIAGNOSED

Fortunately, Lonnie went to the doctor before his cancer had spread. His doctor told him he was very lucky—it's very rare for lung cancer to be detected early. The doctor prescribed surgery to remove Lonnie's cancer.

In addition, Lonnie started making changes in his lifestyle: First, he quit smoking, which wasn't as simple to do as he thought it would be. Instead of being hooked on cocaine, marijuana, crack, or heroin, he was hooked on nicotine.

Lonnie figured he was probably doing other things that put him at risk for the disease, so he requested information from the American Cancer Society (ACS). You'll find the address for ACS in this chapter's Resources section.

Each year, approximately 45,000 black Americans die from a smoking-related disease that could have been prevented. Smoking is a special problem among young black people. According to the Surgeon General's Report *Tobacco Use Among U.S. Racial/Ethnic Minority Groups,* "if current patterns continue, an estimated 1.6 million African Americans who are now under the age of 18 will become regular smokers [and] about 500,00 of those smokers will die of a smoking related disease."[3] That's why eliminating smoking among young people should be a priority.

Although the percentage of people who smoke is decreasing each year, approximately 47 million American adults still smoke, and 25.8 percent of them are black.[4] If you smoke, stop. (For more information about how to quit smoking, see Chapter 2.)

LUNG CANCER

Singer and jazz pianist Nat "King" Cole began his career in the late 1930s as the leader of the King Cole Trio. Later, his velvet voice made him a musical legend. Cole, one of the first blacks successfully to cross over and appeal to white audiences, realized late in his life the dangers of smoking and tried to warn others. James Haskins and Kathleen Benson write, in Cole's biography, that he "talked about how important it was to warn children against smoking and expressed interest in doing advertisements for the American Cancer Society." Cole, a smoker, died from lung cancer shortly after making the statement.

Smoke irritates the lining of your bronchi (the main airways of your lungs), which can cause the cilia (hair-like structures that filter the air entering the lungs) to disappear. Extra mucus, produced to make up for the lack of cilia, causes the coughing that most smokers experience. If you have a persistent cough, blood-streaked sputum, chest pain, or recurring pneumonia or bronchitis, see your doctor immediately. If you're diagnosed with cancer, your doctor can work with you to determine the most appropriate treatment. (For more information on how to break yourself of addictions, see Chapter 2 on taking control, and Chapter 10 on substance abuse.)

PREVENTION AND EARLY DETECTION

Lung cancer, as we've mentioned before, is a very common cancer among black males. But there are many forms of cancer, often with unique methods of prevention and recommended treatment. Eating a high-fiber and low-fat diet, exercising regularly, and reducing stress levels are simple ways you can prevent or control the spread of most cancers. In specific types of the dis-

STEPS YOU CAN TAKE TO LOWER YOUR RISK OF CANCER

To lower your risk of cancer you must watch what you eat and what you do. Here are some of the steps you can take to cut down your chances of getting cancer:

- Eat less fat by choosing lean meats over fatty ones, and by cutting down on butter, margarine, fried foods and rich deserts.
- Eat a variety of vegetables and fruits every day.
- Eat foods high in fiber every day. Good choices include whole grain breads, cereals and pasta, rice, dry beans, fruits and vegetables.
- Cut down on smoked and salt-cured meat like ham, bacon, hot dogs.
- Go easy on alcohol, if you drink.
- Watch your weight. Exercise daily.
- Cover up when the sun is hottest (10 a.m-3 p.m)
- If you work with or near chemicals, wear the right clothes and follow directions exactly.

TOP FIVE CANCER INCIDENT SITES: BLACK MALES

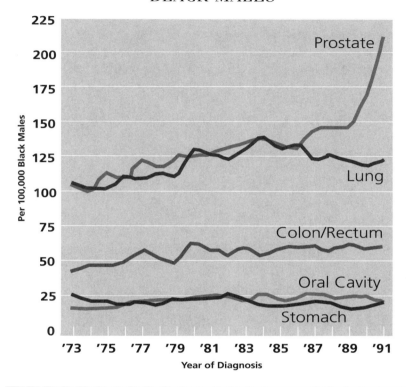

Reprinted with permission of American Cancer Society, "Cancer Incidence in the U.S. 1973-91."

ease, as you'll see, these prevention methods can be especially effective.

Early detection also greatly increases your chance of being cured, so watch your body closely, every day, for any changes that may indicate a problem. In the early stages of many cancers, you may not experience any symptoms at all because many of them don't appear until the disease is more advanced. Because of that, it's important to see your doctor for regular checkups.

Some of cancer's warning signs can include:

1. Change in bowel or bladder habits

2. A sore throat that doesn't heal

3. Unusual bleeding or discharge from the genital, urinary, or digestive tract

4. Thickening or a lump in a breast or elsewhere

5. Indigestion or difficulty swallowing

6. Obvious change in a wart or mole

7. Nagging cough or hoarseness

If you notice any of these symptoms, consult your physician immediately.

OTHER COMMON CANCERS IN BLACK MALES

Many cancers are common among black men. Following are some of these, beginning with those with the highest rates of related deaths for black males in the United States. If you or a loved one wants to prevent or cure a specific cancer, become as educated as possible so that you are fully armed against the disease. See this chapter's Resources section for more information about various forms of cancer.

PROSTATE CANCER

Incidence: Although all men are at risk, prostate cancer is a especially common cancer among black men. In 1999, there were an

INCIDENCE AND MORTALITY RATES* BY SITE, RACE, AND ETHNICITY, UNITED STATES, 1900-1996

Incidence	White	Black	Asian/Pacific Islander	American Indian	Hispanic†
All sites					
Males	480.2	598.0	325.5	177.8	326.9
Females	351.6	335.6	244.9	136.8	243.2
Total	402.9	442.9	279.1	153.4	275.4
Breast (female)	113.2	99.3	82.6	33.9	69.4
Colon & Rectum					
Males	53.2	58.1	47.5	21.5	35.7
Females	36.8	44.9	31.4	12.4	24.0
Total	43.9	50.4	38.6	16.4	29.0
Lung & bronchus					
Males	73.1	112.3	52.4	25.3	38.8
Females	43.3	46.2	22.5	13.5	19.6
Total	55.9	73.9	35.8	18.6	27.6
Prostate	147.3	222.9	81.5	46.5	102.8

Mortality	White	Black	Asian/Pacific Islander	American Indian	Hispanic†
All sites					
Males	208.8	308.8	129.2	123.3	131.8
Females	139.8	168.1	83.5	90.2	86.3
Total	167.5	223.4	103.4	104.0	104.9
Breast (female)	25.7	31.4.	11.4	12.3	15.3
Colon & Rectum					
Males	21.5	27.8	13.4	11.0	13.2
Females	14.5	20.0	9.0	8.9	8.4
Total	170.4	23.1	10.9	9.9	10.4

continued on the next page

"Incidence and Mortality Rates," continued

Mortality	White	Black	Asian/Pacific Islander	American Indian	Hispanic†
Lung & bronchus					
Males	70.1	100.8	34.9	40.5	32.0
Females	33.8	32.8	14.9	19.8	11.0
Total	49.3	60.5	23.7	28.8	19.9
Prostate	23.7	54.8	10.7	14.3	16.7

* Per 100,000, age-adjusted to the 1970 US standard population.

† Hispanic is not mutually exclusive from being a member of another ethnic group.

Note: Incidence data are from the 11 SEER areas; mortality data, except data for Hispanics, are from all states; data for Hispanics include deaths that occured in all states except Connecticut, Louisiana, New Hampshire, and Oklohoma.

Source: US Mortality 1973–1996, National Center for Health Statistics, Centers for Disease Control and Prevention 1999, SEER Incidence 1973°1996, Surveillance, Epidemiology, and End Results Program, Division of Cancer Control and Population Sciences, National Cancer Institute.

Reprinted with permission from the American Cancer Society, "Cancer Facts and Figures 2000, p. 27.

estimated 18,500 new cases of prostate cancer among black men, and in the same year, 6,100 black men were expected to die of the disease.[5] Black men are at least 50 percent more likely to develop prostate cancer and are more than twice as likely to die from it as are men of any other racial and ethnic group.[6]

Those are reasons why you must pay close attention to the prevention and early detection strategies mentioned here: Never delay an annual checkup, and never hesitate to ask your doctor all the questions you may have about this cancer.

We don't know whether the high rate of prostate cancer among black Americans is due to genetic or environmental factors. Some medical experts suggest that eating a high-fat diet may contribute to this disease. Others argue that more black men suffer from this disease than whites because of differences in access to medical care, early detection, and awareness of treatment strategies.

Prevention: Research shows that a diet containing very little alcohol and loaded with lots of fruits and vegetables—especially tomatoes—may help prevent this cancer.

Warning signs: Symptoms include weak or interrupted urine flow; difficulty urinating; the need to urinate frequently; pain in the lower back, pelvis, or upper thighs; blood in urine; and painful ejaculations.

Detection: Every man over age 40 should have a digital rectal examination, which can help detect prostate cancer early, as part of his regular annual physical checkup. Further, at age 50, all men should have an annual prostate-specific antigen (PSA) blood test. If the results of either of these tests seem suspicious, a technique known as transrectal ultrasound can be used to reveal cancers that are too small to be detected through a physical exam.

Treatment: Doctors often use surgery and radiotherapy to treat this cancer. Doctors can now reduce a person's male hormone levels by injecting medications that may also be helpful.

COLORECTAL CANCER

Incidence: In 1999, the American Cancer Society (ACS) estimated that there would be 6,800 new cases of colon and rectal cancer among black men. In the same year, 3,200 black men were expected to die of these diseases.[7] Black men have the highest incidence of colon and rectal cancers and also have higher mortality rates of these cancers than any other racial or ethnic group.[8] As these statistics show, being black seems to have a great effect on whether or not you will survive these cancers.

Prevention: A high-fiber diet, including fruits, grains, and vegetables, can help prevent colon cancer. (Fiber reduces the concentration of carcinogens in your colon because bowel movements are more frequent.) People who take aspirin may also have a lower rate of colon cancer.

Warning signs: Any change in bowel habits, rectal bleeding, and blood in the stool are symptoms.

Detection: After age 40, ask your doctor for a digital rectal exam, stool blood test, and rectum and lower-colon exam (called a flexible sigmoidoscopy) every three or five years. If you are over 50, talk to your doctor about getting a colonoscopy, in which a lighted instrument (called a colonoscope) is inserted into your rectum to view the entire colon. Most insurance companies will pay for this expensive examination only if you're having symptoms.

Treatment: Surgery, with or without chemotherapy, can be an effective treatment for this cancer, depending on the specific location of the cancer and its stage.

ESOPHAGEAL CANCER

Incidence: In 1999, the American Cancer Society estimated that 1,000 new cases of esophageal cancer would be reported among black men and that 1,300 black men would die of the disease that same year.[9] This cancer is about three times more common among African Americans than among whites.[10] The difference in the traditional diets of blacks and whites may be one cause for this inequality, but tobacco smoke and alcohol are the predominant causes.

Prevention: To prevent this cancer, *avoid alcohol, stop smoking,* and reduce the amount of fatty, processed foods you eat. Eat a balanced diet, full of fresh fruits and vegetables. Obesity may contribute to one type of esophageal cancer, so exercise and diet are both important.

Warning signs: Symptoms can include difficulty swallowing or a brief pain behind the breastbone or esophageal area when you swallow.

Detection: A special x-ray called a barium swallow can be used to detect cancer of the esophagus. This procedure involves drinking a chalk-like liquid that contains barium, which coats the esophagus walls and allows your physician to see the esophagus more clearly. Your doctor may also place a gastroscope (tube) down your throat to help detect a cancer.

Treatment: Several treatments are commonly used for cancer of the esophagus, depending on its stage. Surgery is the most common, but doctors substitute chemotherapy and radiotherapy in some cases.

PANCREATIC CANCER

Incidence: In 1999, 1,800 new cases of pancreatic cancer were expected to be reported, while in the same year, experts estimated that 1,500 black men would die of the disease.[11] According to the National Cancer Institute, the incidence of and mortality from this cancer among black men and women are about 50 percent higher than the rates for whites. Among blacks ages 55 to 69, incidence rates exceed those for whites by about 60 percent.[12] These inequalities may stem from differences in traditional diets among blacks and whites, and lifestyle habits, such as the tendency among blacks to smoke more menthol cigarettes than whites.

Prevention: Don't smoke; eat a high-fiber, low-fat diet.

Warning signs: Symptoms may not occur until the cancer is in advanced stages. Warning signals include jaundice, abdominal pain, which may spread to the back, a loss of appetite, nausea, and drastic weight loss or weakness.

Detection: Ultrasound imaging and computerized tomography (CT) scans are sometimes used to detect the disease earlier. Experts know little about what causes this cancer.

Treatment: Doctors often use chemotherapy, radiotherapy, and surgery to treat pancreatic cancer.

Stomach Cancer

Incidence: In 1999, an estimated 1,800 new cases of stomach cancer would be reported among black men, and approximately 1,300 black men would die of the disease.[13]

Prevention: Avoid cured and preserved foods with nitrates, such as hot dogs, beef jerky, and smoked and aged meats.

Warning signs: Loss of appetite, heartburn, stomach pain, or feeling full early in a meal can be signs of stomach cancer. If symptoms last for longer than one month, consult your physician.

Detection: It can be difficult to detect stomach cancer early.

Treatment: Doctors commonly remove all or part of the stomach to treat this cancer; if it has spread, they may also use chemotherapy.

ORAL AND PHARYNGEAL CANCER

Incidence: In 1999, there would be an estimated 2,500 new cases of oral cancer among black men, and approximately 1,000 black men would die of the disease.[14] In fact, according to the National Cancer Institute, the highest incidence or oral cancers is among black men.[15] These inequalities may stem from differences in traditional diets among blacks and whites, and lifestyle habits, such as smoking menthol cigarettes and drinking alcohol.

Prevention: Avoid alcohol. Don't smoke or use chewing tobacco; work to ensure that your home and work environments are smoke-free.

Warning signs: Signs of oral cancer are sores or lumps that may bleed easily and don't heal, and difficulty swallowing and chewing.

Detection: Make sure you have regular checkups with your dentist and doctor. Abnormal tissue changes can often be detected during regular examinations. You may need to have a biopsy if your health care professional finds anything suspicious looking.

Treatment: If cancer is confined to single areas, such as the tongue, lips, or gums, 76 percent can be treated successfully, with a five-year or greater survival rate. If the cancer has spread, though, this number drops to 34 percent. Both surgery and radiation therapy can cure oral cancers, depending on the area(s) involved.

LEUKEMIA

Incidence: In 1999, an estimated 1,100 new cases of leukemias were expected to be reported among black men, and approximately 800 black men would die of these diseases.[16]

Prevention: Prior exposure to radiation or paint removers containing benzene increases the risk of developing leukemia.

Warning signs: Weight loss, repeated infections, fatigue, unusual paleness, bruising easily, and nosebleeds or hemorrhages are common symptoms.

Detection: Symptoms can be similar to those of less serious conditions. Blood tests and biopsy of the bone marrow can determine if what you have is actually leukemia.

Treatment: Chemotherapy is the primary therapy for leukemia. For some types of the disease, your doctor may recommend a bone marrow transplant from a matched donor.

LYMPHOMA

Incidence: According to the ACS, there would be an estimated 3,600 new cases of non-Hodgkin's lymphoma among black men in 1999, and 900 black men would die from it.[17]

Prevention: Risk factors for lymphomas are largely unknown, and the incidence of this disease is increasing. What we do know is that if for any reason you experience reduced immune function (due to an organ transplant, for example) or have been exposed to certain infectious agents, you may be at increased risk. You also may be at increased risk of lymphoma if you have HIV—the AIDS virus. (See Chapter 9 for tips on how to prevent the virus.)

Warning signs: Symptoms of lymphoma are enlargement of lymph nodes, including the spleen, but there's usually no tenderness or pain. Lymph nodes are present in many areas in your body, including your neck, groin, and the area under your arms.

Detection: A biopsy is required to make a diagnosis. Any lymph node larger than 1 inch for more than six weeks should be brought to your physician's attention.

Treatment: Physicians have used chemotherapy and radiation therapy to treat lymphoma; localized lymphomas can frequently be cured with radiation treatments. Some advanced lymphomas are curable with chemotherapy.

CANCER TREATMENTS

Common cancer treatments are surgery, radiation therapy, and chemotherapy. Hormonal therapies may include anti-estrogens, such as tamoxifen or leutenizing hormone reduction injections. New biological treatments include interferon and monoclonal antibodies for breast cancer and lymphoma. In addition to these treatments, many nonmedical alternative therapies are being researched by the medical community, including radical diet changes, positive imaging, increased exercise, as well as humor and relaxation techniques. These complementary therapies may be helpful, but should be used in conjunction with, *not as substitutes for*, traditional therapies. Often, a patient's greatest chance of cure may include a combination of several of these treatments.

Once doctors confirm your diagnosis, it is up to you (with help from your doctor, family members, and trusted love ones) to determine your next move. Since your treatment is a joint venture between you and your doctor, it's important that you take an active role in any health-related decisions and that you ask your doctor to explain the risks and benefits of each treatment he or she recommends. Never hesitate to seek a second opinion.

TREATING CANCER WITH SURGERY

The oldest treatment for cancer is surgery. A surgeon removes cancerous cell growths while cutting away as little healthy tissue as possible. Surgery is a delicate treatment: if your surgeon removes too much healthy tissue, you may suffer from complications. On the other hand, if the surgeon removes too little cancer, you may not be cured. Discuss any proposed surgery with the surgeon who will perform the operation.

Surgeons can remove only those cancers that are confined to a tumor site or regional lymph nodes; if the cancer has spread throughout your body or to your vital organs, you may need to explore other treatment options. All cancer patients must have periodic checkups for the rest of their lives. The cancer-free period associated with "cure" varies for each type of cancer and may be as short as 2 years or as long as 10 years.

TREATING CANCER WITH RADIATION THERAPY

In order to destroy certain cancer cells, your doctor may also use highly active, invisible beams of energy called gamma rays or photons. Radiation may be produced by machines, called linear accelerators, and gamma rays are given off by radioactive substances, such as cobalt, cesium, iridium, and radium. When doctors use radiation to treat cancer, the radioactive substances are usually delivered by a large machine—the linear accelerator. Occasionally, a small container (or needles) containing a radioactive substance are inserted into one of your body cavities or put directly into a tumor.

Although patients can neither see nor feel radiation, this therapy cures cancer by destroying cancer cells. Some cancers are more sensitive than normal tissue to the destructive effects of radiation, such as cancer of the lymph nodes, testicular cancer, and childhood cancers. In these cases, the doctor must irradiate cancer cells in large parts of the body without causing excessive damage to normal tissue.

Radiation is generally used only when the area to be treated is small and confined to one location. When cancer becomes widespread, radiation can seldom produce a cure although it may be used to alleviate the symptoms that accompany cancer. Radiation treatment is also used to treat cancers that can't be surgically removed or cancers that are best not removed because they're vital to the patient's normal activities, such as in the vocal cords and tongue. In other cases, when your doctor is concerned that surgery may leave some cancer cells behind, radiation therapy may be used afterward.

As with any treatment, don't rush into radiation therapy until your doctor has answered all of your questions and concerns, and has designed a program targeted to meet your individual needs. Since radiation may damage some of your healthy cells along with your cancerous cells, it's your doctor's task to destroy the cancer with a minimum of injury to your normal tissues. Because normal cells can repair themselves more efficiently than cancer cells, radiation sessions are spaced so that your healthy cells have time to heal.

If you're undergoing radiation therapy, you may experience some side effects in the area of the body being treated. For example, if your throat is being treated, you may experience a sore throat and have difficulty swallowing; if your bladder or rectum is being treated, you may experience frequent urination, cramps, or diarrhea; if your stomach is being treated, you may feel nauseous. In most instances, though, your doctor can control these side effects with medication.

Radiation of the ovaries or testes can cause infertility, and may cause new cancers several years later, though this happens rarely. The success of radiation therapy can't be determined by the speed at which a tumor shrinks. Slow-growing tumors shrink slowly, whereas fast-growing tumors shrink quickly.

TREATING CANCER WITH CHEMOTHERAPY

When doctors use medications to fight cancer, it's called *chemother-apy*. During chemotherapy, doctors administer one or more anti-cancer drugs in periodic sessions. Each anticancer drug works dif-ferently: One drug, for example, may kill cancer cells by disrupting the process of cell division, whereas another may prevent cells from making the nutrients that keep them alive, and still another may create hormonal conditions in your body that will not allow the cancer cells to survive. Chemotherapy is often used when cancerous cells have spread throughout your body and when doctors can't precisely pinpoint their locations. Unlike surgery and radiation therapy, drugs can circulate throughout your entire body, killing the cancer cells other treatments may miss.

Some cancers, including acute leukemia, lymphoma, and pla-cental and testicular cancers, can be cured by drugs alone. For other types of cancers, such as lung and esophageal cancers, radi-ation plus chemotherapy may cure the disease when neither ther-apy alone is successful. Even when drugs can't produce a cure, though, chemotherapy may still be useful. Chemotherapy may extend a patient's life by making a tumor more responsive to radiation therapy. Chemotherapy drugs may also be used for "adjuvant chemotherapy" after surgery. In that case, doctors use them as a precaution when they're not sure whether some cancer still remains (this is most common in breast cancer and colon cancer). The drugs are intended to destroy cancerous cells that may be alive—but undetected—in the body.

Chemotherapy can be administered in several ways. Some drugs need to be given orally; others must be injected into a vein or under the skin. Doctors have injected chemotherapy into arteries and, if necessary, into the space surrounding the spinal cord. When a single drug can be administered in several ways, the doctor will choose the way best suited to the particular cancer, the prescribed dosage, and your comfort. Health care providers can administer chemotherapy weekly, bimonthly, or monthly and, for short periods of time, daily. Usually, patients can receive their chemotherapy treatments as out-patients, but sometimes they need to be hospitalized.

Like all treatments, chemotherapy has its limitations. If you choose it, make sure your doctor explains the side effects. Because the drugs used may kill normal cells while acting on the cancerous ones, tissues may be damaged, especially those that are made of frequently dividing cells, such as the stomach and intestines, mucous membranes, hair follicles, and bone marrow. Sometimes chemotherapy patients experience nausea, vomiting, and diarrhea (from damage to the digestive tract); mouth dryness and soreness (from mucous membrane damage); and hair loss (from damage to the hair follicles). When bone marrow is damaged, the marrow no longer supplies the blood with the necessary white blood cells, platelets, and red blood cells, so the body can't properly control infection, bruising, or fatigue. Certainly, if you suffer severe side effects from chemotherapeutic treatment, you should work with your physician to have the therapy adjusted. Several new medications are effective in preventing some of these chemotherapy side effects.

LONNIE FINDS LIFE AFTER CANCER

Since Lonnie's diagnosis, he's made some major changes in his lifestyle. He's stopped smoking, eats healthy foods, and exercises regularly. These changes weren't all easy, but if you ask him, he'll tell you that they were all well worth the effort. It's been five years since his surgery. Though Lonnie still goes to the doctor for regular checkups, his doctor reassures him that he has had no recurrence of cancer.

CONCLUSION

As Lonnie learned, it's never too late to quit smoking or to eat a healthier diet. Even though cancer is often curable, it's best to prevent it in the first place by making these lifestyle changes now. Truth is, cancer prevention is only one of the benefits of leading a healthy lifestyle. By cutting down on fat, cholesterol, calories, and salt, and by exercising regularly, you'll not only boost your immune system against disease, you'll feel better every day.

RESOURCES

American Cancer Society
1599 Clifton Road, N.E.
Atlanta, GA 30329
(800) ACS-2345 (800-227-2345)
http://www.cancer.org
(The Society offers information, programs, and patient services.)

American Lung Association
1740 Broadway
New York, NY 10019
(212) 315-8700
(800) LUNG-USA (800-586-4872)
http://www.lungusa.org
(The Association offers general information about lung cancer and how to quit smoking.)

Cancer Fax
(National Cancer Institute)
(301) 402-5874

(Fax your request for information about all different types of cancer and their treatment to this number; your request will be fulfilled by fax.)

Cancer Research Institute
681 Fifth Avenue
New York, NY 10022
(800) 99-CANCER (800-992-2623)
http://www.cancerresearch.org/
(You can receive information about and referrals to cancer studies by calling this 800 number. They will also answer questions and provide literature about your specific areas of interest.)

National Cancer Institute
9000 Rockville Pike
Building 31
Bethesda, MD 20892
(800) 4-CANCER (800–422–6237)
(800) 332–8615 (TTY)
http://www.nci.nih.gov
(The Institute offers patient information and free brochures about diet, cancer prevention, and treatment.)

Office on Smoking and Health
Centers for Disease Control and Prevention
National Center for Chronic Disease Prevention and Health Promotion
Publications Catalog, Mail Stop K-50
4770 Buford Highway, N.E.
Atlanta, GA 30341-3724

(770) 488-5705
(800) CDC-1311
http://www.cdc.gov/tobacco/oshresfa.htm
(This group offers information about tobacco control and statistics about quitting smoking.)

NOTES FOR CHAPTER 6

1. Chinni, Madeline, "Menus for the Anticancer Diet," *Science Digest*, vol. 102, February 1994, p. 14.
2. American Cancer Society, "Cancer Facts and Figures 2000: Graphical Data."
3. "Tobacco Use Among U.S. Racial/Ethnic Minority Groups," A Report of the Surgeon General, U.S. Department of Health and Human Services, Centers for Disease Control and Prevention, National Center for Chronic Disease Prevention and Health Promotion, Office on Smoking and Health, 1998.
4. American Lung Association Fact Sheet, "Smoking," 1999.
5. American Cancer Society, "Cancer Facts and Figures for African Americans," 1998–1999, p. 4.
6. American Cancer Society, Cancer Facts and Figures 2000: "Cancer in Minorities."
7. American Cancer Society, "Cancer Facts and Figures for African Americans," 1998–1999, p. 4.
8. American Cancer Society, Cancer Facts and Figures 2000: "Cancer in Minorities."
9. American Cancer Society, "Cancer Facts and Figures for African Americans," 1998–1999, p. 4.
10. American Cancer Society, The Esophagus Cancer Resource Center, "Esophagus Cancer—Overview," 1999.
11. American Cancer Society, "Cancer Facts and Figures for African Americans," 1998–1999, p. 4.
12. National Cancer Institute, CancerNet, "Pancreas."
13. American Cancer Society, "Cancer Facts and Figures for African Americans," 1998–1999, p. 4.
14. Ibid.
15. National Cancer Institute, CancerNet, "Oral Cavity."
16. American Cancer Society, "Cancer Facts and Figures for African Americans," 1998–1999, p. 4.
17. Ibid.

SEVEN

Sickle Cell Disease

FLETCHER'S STORY

Fletcher is a husky, dark-skinned 35-year-old man with a smile so wide that his face seems to disappear when he's really happy. He works in his local hospital delivering flowers for the florist. He loves his job because he is responsible for delivering a little bit of happiness into sick people's lives. If the patient he's visiting is awake, he never leaves without saying a few kind words. And if one of them seems especially lonely, he always takes time out of his busy day to sit down and start a conversation. Fletcher takes his job very seriously. If he thinks he can make a difference in one of the patients' lives, his secret is not to give up, always to persevere. He learned this technique early in his life, when he suffered his first bout with sickle cell anemia as a child.

WHAT IS SICKLE CELL DISEASE?

Sickle cell disease is a family of inherited blood disease, such as HbSS, SC, SD, SBetaThal. It is sometimes known as sickle cell

NORMAL AND SICKLE CELL

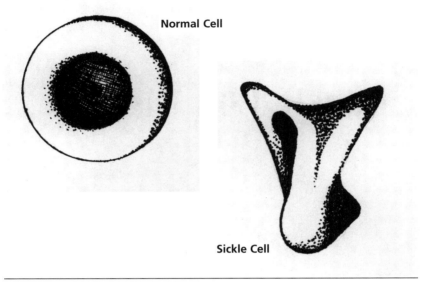

Reprinted with permission of the March of Dimes, from "Public Health Information Sheet, Genetic Series, Sickle Cell Anemia."

anemia, which is HbSS. Red blood cells, when seen under the microscope, are normally round. When you have sickle cell anemia, many of your cells will have a different shape—they look like a crescent moon or a farmer's sickle. These odd-shaped cells are called sickle cells, and the disease they cause is sickle cell anemia.

Red blood cells carry hemoglobin molecules, which transport oxygen from your lungs throughout your body. If you have the sickle cell disease, your hemoglobin molecules stick together after they release the oxygen. This sticking together, combined with the loss of oxygen, causes your hemoglobin molecules to form long, rigid rods inside your red blood cells.

You can be affected by sickle cell hemoglobin in one of two ways: Either you can be "trait carrying" or you can actually have the disease. If you're trait carrying, you usually don't have the symptoms of sickle cell disease (mentioned later in this chapter), but you can pass the trait on to your children, just as one of your parents passed the sickle cell trait to you. For example, civil rights leader Jesse Jackson carries the trait for sickle cell disease but is, obviously, very healthy. If you *have* the disease, on the other hand, you'll most likely experience many of the symptoms we'll discuss later in this chapter, and may need regular medical care.

If you have the disease, not only do some of your red blood cells become sickle shaped, but your red blood cells can lose their flexibility, which makes it more difficult for them to pass through small blood vessels. These cells, which are now oddly shaped and sticky, can clog your small blood vessels, causing your healthy red blood cells to become stuck behind them. Whatever organ or tissue this clogged vessel leads to is deprived of an adequate blood supply. Such blockages cause most of the problems and pain that accompany sickle cell disease. Furthermore, the life span of red blood cells, when "sickled," is shortened to 10 to 20 days, whereas normal cells live about 130 days. As a result, bone marrow can't make cells quickly enough, resulting in profound anemia (low red blood count).

Two myths surround sickle cell disease. One is that it's contagious. The truth is, you cannot catch sickle cell disease from another person. The second myth is that people with the disease do not live past the age of 20. This is also false. Many people with sickle cell disease live to enjoy old age. In severe cases, though, people can die as children or young adults.

HOW DO I KNOW IF I AM A CANDIDATE FOR SICKLE CELL DISEASE?

As we mentioned, sickle cell disease is an inherited disease. Here's how it works: If both of your parents are trait carriers, and both parents passed a sickle cell hemoglobin gene on to you, then you will have sickle cell disease. If your parents passed the gene for sickle cell disease to you, it can have many different implications for your children.

- If you carry the sickle cell trait (SA), and your partner has normal hemoglobin (AA), you have a 50 percent chance of conceiving a child with normal hemoglobin (AA) and a 50 percent chance of having a child who carries the sickle cell trait (SA). There is no chance that any of your children will actually have the disease.

- If you have sickle cell disease (SS) and your partner has normal hemoglobin (AA), all the children you conceive will carry the sickle cell trait (SA); none of them will be born with normal hemoglobin (AA). But the good news is that none of your children will actually have sickle cell disease (SS).

- If both you and your partner carry the sickle cell trait (SA), you have a 25 percent chance of having a child with normal hemoglobin (AA); a 50 percent chance of conceiving a child who carries the sickle cell trait (SA); and a 25 percent chance of having a child with sickle cell disease (SS).

- If you carry the trait for sickle cells (SA) and your partner has the disease (SS), you have a 50 percent chance of having a child who carries the trait (SA), and a 50 percent chance of conceiving a child with sickle cell disease (SS).

- If both you and your partner have sickle cell disease (SS), all of your children will have the disease as well (SS).

- If neither you nor your partner carries the trait or has the disease (AA), there is no chance that any of your children will have sickle cell disease.

- Certain hemoglobin traits can combine with sickle hemoglobin to cause cell diseases such as Hemoglobin C, D, and Beta thalassemia.

Years ago, if both partners carried the trait for sickle cell disease, or had the disease, it was common for doctors to discourage such a couple from having children. Today, doctors will generally inform parents-to-be of the complications their child may encounter, but whether or not the couple chooses to have a child will be left up to them.

WHAT ARE THE SIGNS AND SYMPTOMS OF SICKLE CELL DISEASE?

The primary symptom of sickle cell disease is pain brought on by a sickle cell crisis, or a blockage in a blood vessel. If you have the disease, you may feel pain anywhere in your body and at any time. (The intensity and frequency of episodes varies with each person.) Fletcher, for example, averages one or two incidents of pain each year; you may have more or less frequent occurrences. The intensity of your pain may also vary. Sometimes, if you have sickle cell disease, the pain can be so intense that you need to be hospitalized, but that's only necessary until your pain subsides and the crisis in your blood is resolved.

Dactylitis

Dactylitis, or Hand Foot Syndrome, can occur in babies and children with sickle cell disease. It causes painful swelling of the hands and feet. Such swellings are one of the first complications in sickle cell syndromes, with the highest incidence between ages six months and two years. Doctors treat the condition with fluids and pain medication. It usually will go away within a few days without further problems.

Stroke

Strokes are more common in children with sickle cell disease. A special ultrasound test, the Trans Cranial Doppler, or TCD, can detect which children are at high risk for stroke. Monthly blood transfusions can prevent the first stroke, and it is the only treatment, after a stroke had occurred, that will prevent another. Any new weakness, numbness, trouble talking, or facial droop should be checked by a physician immediately.

Sequestration

Sequestration is the clogging of sickled red cells in the spleen or liver. This can cause swelling in the abdomen or general weakness. Sequestration is an *emergency* and requires immediate hospitalization and treatment with blood transfusions. Sometimes a surgeon must remove your spleen to keep this from recurring.

Infections

Infections are more common in sickle cell patients because their spleens don't work to protect them from germs. All children who have the disease should take daily penicillin from birth to age six to prevent deadly infections from the germ pneumococcus. A sickle cell patient with a fever should be seen by a doctor immediately. Patients should not try to make the fever go away on their own with any fever-reducing medication (such as acetaminophen, ibuprofen, or aspirin) until their doctor says it's okay to do so.

Anemia

Anemia is a common consequence of the disease—hence the name sickle cell "anemia." Anemia simply means that you have a low blood count or a decrease in your normal level of red blood cells. The sickled cell has a greatly shortened life span (two weeks), compared to the life span of a normal healthy red blood cell (about 130 days).

Bone marrow, which produces your red blood cells, can't keep up with the short lifespan of your sickled cells. If you have anemia, you may experience headache, weakness, dizziness, and nausea; your skin may appear pale.

Jaundice

Another sign of sickle cell disease is jaundice, when the white part of your eyes turns yellowish. This condition, also called *icterisclera,* is usually not painful and may be a sign that blood cells are breaking up within your blood vessels.

Aseptic Necrosis

Aseptic necrosis is the name given to deterioration and loss of bone in the hips or shoulders, secondary to lost or poor blood supply to that area. This condition can often be confused with arthritis, but the pain is usually more severe.

Leg Ulcers

If you have sickle cell disease, poor circulation may cause ulcers to form around your ankles. So if you have been diagnosed with sickle cell disease, pay attention to any sores that seem to be slow in healing, and to chronic swelling of your legs, and show these physical changes to your doctor for advice.

Priapism

Common in young males, priapism occurs when a man gets a painful erection because of cells sickling in the penis. Episodes like this can be caused by prolonged intercourse, masturbation, or infection. Warm baths and immediate bladder emptying may reduce the discomfort or lessen the problem; however, if priapism persists for longer than three hours, seek medical attention for pharmacological intervention.

SICKLE CELL DISEASE AND BLACKS

One in every 10 black Americans carries the sickle cell trait, and an estimated 1 out of every 400 black babies is born in the United States each year with sickle cell disease. Although the disorder affects more blacks than people of other races, some individuals who originate from the Caribbean, Latin America, Mediterranean, Middle East, and Southeast Asia or India also suffer from the disease. Fifty thousand Americans have sickle cell disease, making it a significant health problem in the United States today.

Some experts say that the prevalence of sickle cell disease among blacks is a clue to our African roots. Ironically, there is a survival-of-the-fittest story here. If you have the sickle cell trait, you have a better chance of surviving malaria, a red cell infection. If you were born with sickle cell trait in a country ravaged by malaria, such as Africa or Haiti, you had a greater chance of survival than did many people around you without the sickle cell trait. As a result, in these countries, people with the sickle cell trait survived and grew up to have children who inherited the sickle cell trait. When their children moved away to other areas of the world, they took the disease with them and continued to pass it to future generations.

In certain patients, sickle cell disease can now be cured with bone marrow transplantation, although not every sickle cell patient is a candidate for the procedure. Symptoms of sickle cell disease may be prevented with the medication hydroxyurea.

FLETCHER COPES WITH PAIN

Sometimes Fletcher's pain becomes severe. Since his birth, he has had pain in every part of his body, depending on where his sickled cells happen to clog. He's lucky, though, because he gets the bad pain only once or twice a year. Other people with sickle cell anemia suffer more frequently because they don't practice as many prevention techniques as Fletcher does. Fletcher learned when he was very young how to prevent pain and avoid crises by taking good care of himself. He avoids dehydration and extreme temperatures, and prevents infections—a difficult feat considering that he works at a hospital and spends most of his time visiting sick people.

Usually, Fletcher fends off serious infections by asking his doctor to prescribe antibiotics at their early onset. But every once in a while, an infection will develop that sends his body into a tailspin. If his pain is too bad, Fletcher is admitted to the hospital, where he receives treatment and pain medication until the crisis resolves. That usually takes a few days. Then Fletcher is back at work, without much more than a memory of the pain. He's lucky, and he knows it.

When Fletcher is admitted to the hospital, he usually meets other people with sickle cell anemia, many of whom are there for the fifth, sixth, even the tenth time that year. Fletcher has learned how fortunate he is because his disease is less severe than that of most sickle cell patients, who don't take such good care of themselves. So Fletcher talks to them, and before they know it, he's telling them how they can avoid infection and prevent unnecessary and uncomfortable hospital stays. They can't help listening: Fletcher isn't one to give up easily.

HOW TO AVOID INFECTION

Here are some of the tips that Fletcher usually shares with his newfound friends. Some of them can be very difficult to put into practice all the time, but it's helpful to be aware of what may be leading to their crises.

- Try to stay clear of people with contagious infections such as flu and strep throat.

- If you have an early sign of infection such as a cough, pain during urination, sore throat, or fever, see your doctor immediately. Have a culture taken and ask to be treated with antibiotics, if appropriate. Rest, drink lots of fluids, and ask your doctor about other medications that may help you to recover quickly.

- If you develop a sore, abrasion, or cut on your skin, make sure you seek medical treatment immediately. Also remember to keep the affected area clean.

- If you develop infected cysts or pus pockets, these usually need to be drained. Antibiotics alone may not do the job of clearing these infections.

- Take preventive steps, such as getting flu shots or immunizations or taking preventive medications when traveling to certain countries. The health department is a good resource for information about these measures. Of course, consult your doctor before taking any medication or vaccines. You should get a flu shot every year and a pneumococcal vaccine every 10 years. Children should have the pneumococcal vaccine at ages two and six.

- Avoid extreme temperatures.

- Avoid caffeine and alcohol, and drink plenty of water every day, to limit your chances of becoming dehydrated.

- Children who have the disease should take daily penicillin from birth to age six.

WHAT COMPLICATIONS MIGHT I EXPERIENCE?

Of the symptoms and complications we've discussed, one sickle cell patient may have a few, whereas another may have an entirely different experience with the disease. Only a relatively small percentage of sickle cell patients will experience all the symptoms we've listed.

Most of the complications of sickle cell disease are caused by sickling of your red blood cells, which partially or fully prevents oxygenated blood from reaching your organs. If an artery leading to one of your vital organs is blocked by sickled cells for a long period of time, it can cause irreparable damage.

Though narcotics can lessen the pain you may feel from the blockage, no one has yet discovered a way to prevent the sickling from happening in the first place. The area where the sickling occurs is very important because a blockage in an artery leading to certain areas, such as your brain, can be life threatening. It can also be dangerous to have sickled cells in vital organs such as your heart, liver, kidney, lungs, or eyes for an extended period.

Sometimes people with sickle cell disease suffer damage to their eyes because of the clotting difficulty. Many people with the disease will appear to have yellow eyes. This is caused by the breakdown of red blood cells. Your retina, the part of your eye that provides your brain with information about what you are seeing, is especially sensitive to oxygen and blood losses. If clotting in your retina lasts for a long time, your vision can be irreparably damaged.

It's easy for a health professional to confuse complications that result from sickle cell disease with the symptoms of other diseases. Life-threatening diseases can be misdiagnosed as sickle cell disease, or vice versa. If you know you have sickle cell disease, be sure to tell your doctor so that he or she won't confuse the symptoms of sickle cell disease with other illnesses.

SHOULD I BE TESTED FOR SICKLE CELL DISEASE?

Even if you've never experienced any of the symptoms that we described earlier, as a member of a high-risk minority, you should still be tested for the sickle cell disease. The test, called hemoglobin electrophoresis, is simple and can easily be arranged by your doctor or any health care professional. Hemoglobin electrophoresis will determine whether you carry the sickle cell trait—valuable information for you and your partner if you want to plan a family. In fact, it's a good idea for your whole family to be tested for the sickle cell trait. (In most states, newborns are now being screened for sickle cell disease.)

TREATING THE DISEASE

Bone marrow transplants now offer a cure for sickle cell disease, but they aren't an appropriate treatment for everyone. Complications of the disease can usually be treated with drugs, surgery, antibiotics, pain medication, or simple bed rest. As we mentioned earlier, prevention is crucial. Medications such as hydroxyurea can prevent events from occurring. As Fletcher did, you can lessen the number of episodes you have by taking good care of yourself:

- Try to avoid infections because they can lead to a sickle cell episode. (Read Chapter 2 for more information about how to prevent general diseases and infections.)

- Exercise regularly, but not too strenuously.

- Eat a proper diet and drink at least eight glasses of water every day. Extra fluids can help your body ward off a sickle cell crisis.

- Avoid temperature extremes—either too hot or too cold—and get enough rest

- Try to avoid stress whenever possible.

- When you have to stay in bed for a prolonged period, use an incentive spivomenter (commonly known as a "blow bottle") to prevent chest syndrome, or sickling in the lungs.

CONCLUSION

If you have sickle cell disease, take the time to learn about your disease and how best to cope with its complications. Follow the guidelines outlined in this book, use common sense, and listen to what your body is telling you. By following these simple tips, like Fletcher, you, too, can benefit from a healthier life.

RESOURCES

Sickle Cell Disease Association of America
200 Corporate Point # 945
Culver City, CA 90230-7633
(800) 421-8453
(310) 216-6363
http://www.sicklecelldisease.org
(The Association will provide you with genetic counseling and brochures; they will refer you to an office in your area for more information and possible financial aid.)

National Heart, Lung, and Blood Institute
Sickle Cell Disease Branch
6701 Rockledge Drive MSC 7950
Bethesda, MD 20892-7950
(301) 435-0055
http://www.nhlbi.nih.gov
(This website offers information on a wide variety of health topics and information on clinical trials.)

**The Georgia Comprehensive Sickle Cell Center at Grady
Health System**
P.O. Box 109
Grady Memorial Hospital
80 Butler St.
Atlanta, GA 30335
(404) 616-3572 (24 hours)
(404) 616-5998 (fax)
http://www.emory.edu/PEDS/SICKLE
*(The Center offers an online tutorial, web links, research news,
and clinical guidelines.)*

EIGHT

Kidney Disease

MARCUS'S STORY

Marcus and his wife own four dry cleaning stores, which employ 50 people. Though he's now 58, Marcus has been working his way up the economic ladder ever since he quit school at age 14 to work at a dry cleaners to help support his family. By the time he turned 20, he was managing a cleaning store and saving his money wisely until he could afford to start his own business. As it turned out, the business he started was such a success that he added three more stores to his chain within eight years.

Marcus, who works hard and talks like a born salesman, also has kidney disease. Since age 45, he has undergone regular dialysis therapy (which uses an artificial kidney to provide the same functions as his original kidneys) because his kidneys have totally shut down. Marcus had some initial difficulty adapting to dialysis because it takes him away from his business three days a week for three-and-a-half hours each time. While he's away, he's often restless and fidgety, worrying about what's going on at his stores. His wife always reassures him the business is fine since his sons run it while he's gone.

WHAT IS KIDNEY (OR RENAL) DISEASE OR KIDNEY FAILURE?

To answer both questions, let's talk first about normal kidney function. Our kidneys have three major duties to help keep us in good health. First, kidneys filter our blood. (This filtering removes waste products from the body.) Second, our kidneys also help our bodies to maintain the proper balance and concentrations of electrolytes, such as potassium and sodium, so they don't become toxic. Finally, kidneys make hormones that help keep our bones strong and prevent anemia. (It's interesting to note that even though we're born with two kidneys, one kidney alone is enough to cleanse the blood adequately and to regulate our body fluids.)

The term *kidney disease* refers to any condition that keeps the kidneys from working properly. (Even seemingly unrelated diseases—diabetes is one example—can lead to kidney disease.) If the kidney damage isn't remedied, it can, over time, lead to kidney failure. The most advanced form of kidney failure is called end stage renal disease, or ESRD.

In case you think you don't need to read this chapter, consider this: Many people think they can't have kidney disease because they still pass a lot of urine, but you can't really tell that way. It's not the amount of urine that you produce that is of concern, but the amount of *waste* that your urine contains that tells doctors how well your kidneys are actually working. (When your kidneys aren't working properly, they contain less waste and more water.)

THE KIDNEYS, URETERS, AND BLADDER

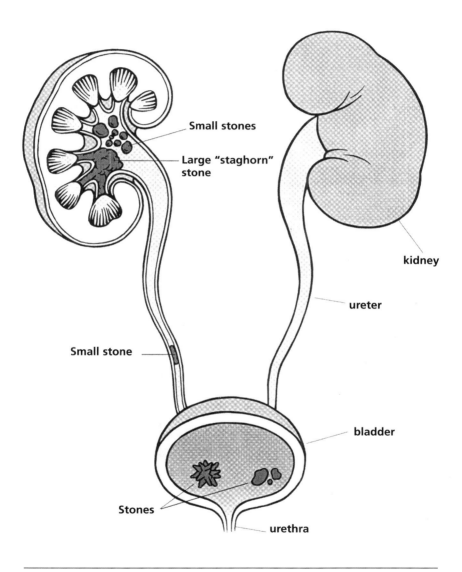

Reprinted with permission from "About Kidney Stones," © 2000, American Cancer Society.

KIDNEY DISEASE IN BLACKS

Kidney failure has become a major public health issue for the black community. Here are the alarming dimensions of the epidemic: Although blacks make up 12 percent of the U.S. population, they account for nearly 30 percent of the patients on dialysis.[1] For example, in Georgia, blacks make up 30 percent of the population but 67 percent of patients with ESRD.[2] Unfortunately, this number is increasing by approximately 10 percent a year.

HOW DO I KNOW IF I HAVE KIDNEY DISEASE?

People with kidney disease may not have symptoms in the disease's early stages because the kidneys are able to compensate for a while. By the time you begin to have symptoms, you may already have lost more than two-thirds of your kidney function. Fortunately, your doctor can use urine and blood tests to detect the early signs of kidney disease.

Urine Tests

For centuries, dating back to the time of Hippocrates, physicians have used urine tests to learn about internal organ disease. (It's hard to believe, but in ancient times, physicians used to taste urine in order to detect diabetes! If you have diabetes, your urine contains excess sugar, so it would taste sweet.) When your kidneys are damaged, the filtering process becomes faulty, causing certain materials to build up in your urine. It's no wonder, then, that your doctor requests a urine sample during your checkup. Here are some of the things your physician looks for in a urinalysis.

- In healthy people, doctors find little or no protein in urine samples. If you have kidney disease, they can detect an increased amount of protein in the urine (proteinuria). In the disease's earliest phase, doctors can detect only very small amounts of a protein called albumin. This condition is called microalbuminuria.

- Too much glucose in your urine can be a sign of diabetes, kidney disease, or both.

- Too much bacteria in the urine may be a sign of kidney or bladder infection.

- Blood or pus in the urine can also be a sign of kidney disease.

- Too little acid or too much acid in your urine can also indicate kidney disease.

The Nitrite Test

You can also test your urine for infection at home by using a nitrite urine-testing kit (available at pharmacies). These kits, which are about 70 percent accurate, contain chemically treated paper strips, which you insert into an early-morning urine sample. The color of the strip changes if there is bacteria-producing nitrite in your urine.

Blood Tests

Some blood tests can tell doctors that your kidneys may not be working properly. These are BUN (blood, urea, nitrogen) and creatinine.

Cystoscopy

During this procedure, your doctor uses an instrument—called a cystoscope—to look into your bladder. The cystoscope has a light source as well as other attachments that can remove stones from your bladder, biopsy suspicious-looking areas, and relieve obstructions. If your doctor performs cystoscopy properly, this procedure should not affect your sexual function.

Ultrasound or Computerized Tomography (CT) Scan

Both of these tests help your doctor assess basic defects or changes in your kidneys. For example, in people with chronic kidney failure, a CT scan detects small, shrunken kidneys. A CT scan also helps doctors exclude a cancer diagnosis in people with bloody urine. Ultrasound tests, on the other hand, may detect kidney stones that can cause pain and bloody urine.

A WORD ABOUT KIDNEY STONES

In some people, certain minerals build up to form hard stones of various shapes and sizes. Problems occur when the stones lodge in areas of the kidney or ureters to block urine flow and cause kidney damage. Stones can cause bloody urine and may lead to urinary infections. Some stones are so small they can pass through your system without too many problems; others, however, can become large enough to make them difficult or impossible to pass and cause excruciating pain.

Kidney stone treatment varies from person to person, depending on the composition and size of the stone; only about 10 percent of all people with kidney stones have to undergo surgery. Usually, your doctor will tell you to drink lots of fluids every day to help pass the stones and to help prevent new ones. (By drinking lots of fluids, you continually dilute your urine and prevent too many concentrated minerals from depositing in your kidneys.) Your doctor may also prescribe medication that both treats and prevents stones. Another way to treat kidney stones is called extracorporeal shock-wave lithostripy (ESWL), which breaks them up using shock waves. Though you should never ignore any symptoms of kidney disease, people with kidney stones do not usually have kidney failure.

KIDNEY FAILURE

There are two types of kidney failure: acute and chronic. In acute kidney failure, the kidneys suddenly stop working properly. For example, if a person has the early stages of kidney disease, resulting from hypertension or a prostate blockage, and then takes a medication that might be safe in most situations—such as ibuprofen—it could trigger kidney failure. You can also suffer from kidney failure if you don't drink enough water when you're training for an athletic event or performing strenuous manual labor. Luckily, appropriate therapy can often reverse acute kidney failure though you may need dialysis for a little while.

Earlier we referred to chronic kidney failure by its other name, ESRD (end stage renal disease). ESRD is irreversible.

WHAT CAUSES KIDNEY FAILURE?

Data from the 1999 United States Renal Data System (USRDS) report shows that there are five major causes of chronic (irreversible) kidney failure in blacks:[3] diabetes; hypertensive renal disease; glomerulonephritis; HIV-associated nephropathy; and interstitial kidney diseases, such as pyelonephritis, polycystic kidney disease, and kidney disease from sickle cell anemia.

For most of these diseases, heredity may play a role. Although researchers can't explain all the genetic factors involved in kidney failure, they do understand those involved in polycystic kidney disease, or PKD. PKD is a disorder in which the kidneys are filled with small balloon-like cysts that progressively increase in size and eventually damage the kidneys. We'll discuss this disorder more fully later in this chapter.

DIABETES

Worldwide, diabetes has become the most common cause of kidney failure. According to data from the 1999 USRDS report, diabetic nephropathy (kidney damage from diabetes) accounted for 39 percent of the cases of ESRD among black patients in the United States.[4] Diabetes is approximately twice as common in blacks as in whites, and diabetic ESRD occurs three to six times more frequently in blacks than in whites.[5]

When diabetes injures your kidneys, they're unable to clean your blood properly. In fact, doctors can tell that a kidney has been injured when they find small amounts of protein in your urine (called microalbuminuria). Over time, kidney damage causes you to leak large amounts of protein into your urine, which often appears with leg swelling, facial puffiness, and worsening blood pressure control. These changes may cause you to go to the bathroom more frequently at night.

As your kidney fails, you may become nauseous and weak, vomit, lose your appetite, itch, and suffer from leg cramps and anemia (low blood count). Some people may notice a bad taste in their mouths, whereas others have urine-scented breath. These are all signs of severe kidney failure, and if you develop such symptoms, you must talk to your doctor about dialysis as soon as possible. Having your diabetes and blood pressure under good control may help to slow the progression of kidney damage. People with diabetes should follow a proper diet (see a registered dietitian or certified diabetes educator for details), avoid smoking, and take insulin or oral blood sugar pills (oral hypoglycemic agents) as prescribed. If your kidneys are spilling protein into your urine, you may be put on a special class of blood pressure pills called ACE inhibitors (angiotensin converting enzyme inhibitor), which can help protect the kidney from the ravages of diabetes.[6]

HYPERTENSIVE RENAL DISEASE

Hypertensive renal disease is the second leading cause of kidney failure in blacks. Data from the 1999 USRDS report shows that hypertensive renal disease accounts for 34.2 percent of all cases of ESRD in blacks[7]. Not only do blacks have an increased incidence of hypertension, they are also 17 times more likely than white patients to get kidney failure as a result of hypertension. Blacks with high blood pressure appear to progress to kidney failure (ESRD) faster than some other races, especially if they have protein in their urine. Research suggests that physicians are more likely to blame hypertension as the cause of kidney failure in black patients without investigating other possibilities.

If you have high blood pressure, you need to take your blood pressure medicines religiously to prevent kidney damage. Untreated or poorly treated hypertension damages the small kidney blood vessels, which causes them to become thick and rigid. This damage to the kidney vessels reduces blood supply to the kidneys and reduces their ability to cleanse the blood properly. This poor filtering, in turn, leads to accumulation of waste products in the body. Keeping your blood pressure under strict control certainly helps prevent kidney disease.

GLOMERULONEPHRITIS

Our kidneys are able to filter the blood with the help of very small blood vessels called glomeruli. People get glomerulonephritis when these vessels are inflamed or destroyed. When these "filters" are damaged, protein and blood leak into the urine. There are two types of glomerulonephritis—acute and chronic. Glomerulonephritis accounted for 8.6 percent of the causes of ESRD in blacks in 1999.

Acute glomerulonephritis occurs more commonly in children. Doctors often find it when they're looking at bloody urine. Other symptoms of this disease include facial puffiness and increased blood pressure. People with this disease may get better all of a sudden, but the high blood pressure that goes along with this illness may cause serious problems.

Chronic glomerulonephritis results when our kidneys are persistently inflamed. This disease may often progress slowly but continuously, and may eventually lead to terminal kidney failure. In unusual cases, the disease may lead to kidney failure quickly— even in as few as three to six months.

The symptoms that accompany chronic glomerulonephritis are few, but you may notice extra white foam in the toilet when you urinate, bloody or cola-colored urine, facial puffiness, ankle swelling, and back pain. And if you've just been diagnosed with high blood pressure, or if your blood pressure becomes hard to control, you should see a doctor to rule out this illness. (Having any of these symptoms doesn't necessarily mean you have this condition, but you should seek medical help immediately to be sure.)

Making changes in your diet can improve some disease. For example, if you have blood pressure along with glomerulonephritis, you should eat less salt. (Ask your doctor to recommend a healthy diet for you.) If your kidneys are severely damaged, you may need dialysis or a kidney transplant.

HIV-ASSOCIATED NEPHROPATHY

An increasing number of inner-city blacks are developing a very aggressive form of glomerulonephritis that's associated with HIV infection, the virus that causes AIDS. Some people with kidney disease and AIDS can develop terminal kidney failure from chronic glomerulonephritis within three to six months. People with HIV infection who get kidney disease can benefit from ACE inhibitors, as well as medicines that directly destroy the virus, such as AZT and other new drugs. In 1999, kidney disease related to HIV infection accounted for 3 percent of ESRD cases among blacks.[8] Unfortunately, kidney failure from AIDS is more common among blacks than whites. If you have symptoms of HIV infection, such as weight loss, fever, or chronic diarrhea, please seek medical attention immediately.

INTERSTITIAL KIDNEY DISEASES

The area of the kidney outside the small vessel clusters (glomeruli) is called the interstitial area. Interstitial diseases can also cause kidney failure.

PYELONEPHRITIS

Sometimes urine can back up from the bladder into our kidneys because of a faulty valve between the bladder and the ureter. When this happens, bacteria in our urine can infect and scar the kidneys—a condition called pyelonephritis. If you experience a burning sensation when you urinate, suffer from chills, fever, or see blood in your urine, you may have pyelonephritis and should seek medical attention immediately. Antibiotics cure this condition if it's treated early, but if you leave it untreated, pyelonephritis can lead to irreversible kidney failure (ESRD).

POLYCYSTIC KIDNEY DISEASE

Polycystic kidney disease, which is hereditary, occurs when cysts or small pockets form in your kidneys, making your kidneys look similar to a cluster of grapes. These cysts gradually enlarge, causing pain, pressure damage to your kidneys, and high blood pressure. People with polycystic kidney disease often pass bloody urine, suffer from back pain, recurrent urinary tract infections, and kidney failure. Though there's currently no cure for this disease, it's important to seek medical attention early if you have any of the symptoms we've mentioned. It's also a good idea to ask your relatives if there's a history of kidney disease in your family.

KIDNEY FAILURE IN SICKLE CELL DISEASE

Sickle cell anemia can also cause kidney failure (see Chapter 7 for full details of sickle cell anemia). A recent report from the USRDS indicated that, between 1992 and 1996, there were 345 new cases of ESRD caused by sickle cell renal disease among people eligible for Medicare in the United States.[9] Studies show that kidney transplantation may offer a survival advantage over dialysis in people with sickle cell kidney failure.[10]

UREMIA

Kidney failure causes uremia. Uremia is the accumulation of body wastes (toxins) that poison your body and have caused your kidneys to fail irreversibly. People with uremia may experience some of the following reactions:

- When your kidneys shut down, they're no longer able to filter and remove potassium from your body. Although optimal levels of potassium can help heart, muscle, and nerve tissue function properly, in people with uremia, too much of this mineral can stop your heart and cause you to die suddenly.

- Healthy kidneys release a hormone called erythropoietin into the blood, which stimulates production of red blood cells. People with uremia have low levels of this hormone, which slows down the production of red blood cells and leads to anemia. If your skin is becoming pale and you feel tired all the time, you may be anemic. Talk to your doctor.

- People with uremia often suffer from hypertension. High levels of sodium in the blood cause retention of fluid in the blood vessels, raising the blood pressure.

- If you suffer from uremia, you may notice skin color changes. Some people may become darker, whereas others become yellowish. (This yellowish tint is not related to jaundice, which is caused by liver disease.) If you have darker skin, you may notice this yellow tint in skin creases or around your eyes; some black men's skin may take on a grayish color. You may also suffer from stubborn itching.

- In the final stages of uremia, your body's poison buildup may cause your nerves to become tranquilized, which could cause you to go into a coma unless you undergo dialysis or an organ transplant.

PREVENTING KIDNEY FAILURE

You can avoid acute kidney failure by avoiding medications that can cause kidney damage and by drinking enough fluid before exposing yourself to potentially damaging substances (such as contrast media dyes and certain antibiotics). Further, you can help to prevent chronic kidney failure by:

- *Controlling your blood pressure.* Increased blood pressure damages kidneys. If you have kidney disease, it is usually best to keep your blood pressure in the 125/75 mm Hg range.

- *Managing your diabetes.* You'll know your diabetes is under control by measuring your blood level of a special type of hemoglobin called glycosylated hemoglobin A_{1c}. For diabetic patients whose kidneys are spilling protein, a special class of antihypertensive medicines called ACE inhibitors has been shown to help prevent or slow the progression to ESRD. These drugs also benefit people who suffer from kidney disease as a result of HIV and sickle cell disease.

- *Eating a healthy diet.* A proper diet is critical for people with diabetes. A low-salt diet is important because it helps to reduce blood pressure. You should discuss your diet thoroughly with your doctor and your dietitian. It's also important for people with diabetes to control their weight and get plenty of exercise.

- *Seeing a kidney specialist.* If you or someone you love is diagnosed with kidney failure, ask your doctor for a referral to a kidney doctor (a nephrologist) as soon as possible.

MARCUS PERSEVERES

Marcus felt as if he were wasting many hours during dialysis that he could have spent working at his stores. But his sons pointed out that he could get a lot of work done during dialysis. Now Marcus takes his accounting books, order forms, and cell phone to dialysis so that he can do business while he's there. He balances the books, places orders, and handles customer and personnel problems all from the dialysis center. Quick with a sales pitch and his business card, Marcus drums up new business from nurses, doctors, and patients alike.

END STAGE RENAL DISEASE (ESRD) AND ITS TREATMENT

Fifty years ago, a diagnosis of ESRD was considered a death sentence. Now, medical advances have made it treatable. The three major therapies are hemodialysis, peritoneal dialysis, and kidney transplantation.

HEMODIALYSIS

Hemodialysis removes accumulated body wastes (toxins), certain minerals, and excess fluid from your body by circulating your blood through an artificial kidney called a dialyzer. Basically, this machine uses a special filter (the dialyzer) to clean your blood and remove unwanted body wastes. Once the blood is cleansed, it is returned to your body through another set of tubes. People on hemodialysis need to undergo treatment at least three times a week, and one session lasts from three to four hours. Patients undergo hemodialysis at a dialysis clinic or center though it can also be done at the patient's home. During treatment, some people may experience nausea, muscle cramps, dizziness, or weakness because their blood pressure can drop suddenly, a condition called hypotension. If you have any of these symptoms during dialysis, report them to your doctor or nurse. While you're on dialysis, try to follow these guidelines:

- Don't miss treatments. If you're body wastes aren't removed, you could get sick. Your doctor will keep track of how long you are dialyzed every month: Too little dialysis can shorten your life.

- Control your diet. Avoid foods rich in potassium (such as bananas), which may raise your potassium to a dangerous level. Large amounts of cheese, milk, and other dairy products may contribute to weakening your bones.

- Watch your fluids. If you drink too much fluid, your blood pressure might go up and make you feel ill during dialysis.

- Control your salt intake. Too much salt raises your blood pressure and can cause heart failure.

HEMODYALISIS.

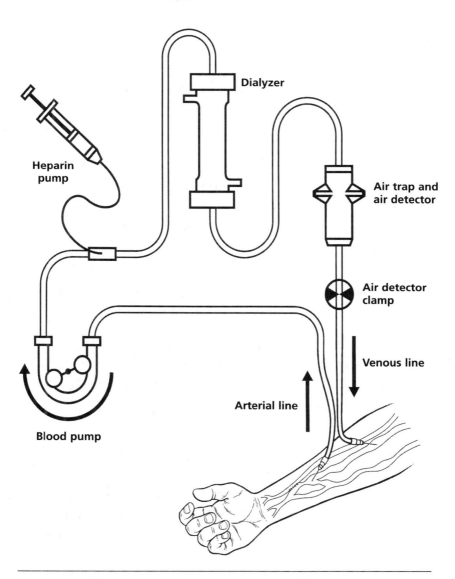

Advances in hemodialysis, such as faster, more efficient filters (dialyzers), mean patients now have an improved—and longer— quality of life.

PERITONEAL DIALYSIS (PD)

Peritoneal dialysis is an alternative form of dialysis that uses part of your own body—the lining of the abdominal cavity or peritoneal membrane—to filter your blood. Doctors place a catheter and a sterile cleansing solution, called dialysate, into your abdominal cavity. (The catheter stays there for as long as you're undergoing peritoneal dialysis.) All of your body's waste products pass into the dialysate from blood vessels in your peritoneal membrane. Health professionals drain the dialysate from your body after a few hours, and introduce fresh dialysate. Then the process begins again.

There are three common forms of peritoneal dialysis:

1. Continuous Ambulatory Peritoneal Dialysis (CAPD). Most people with ESRD use this type of peritoneal dialysis. "Ambulatory" means that the dialysis takes place while you're moving around during the day. No machine is used with this type of dialysis; the dialysate enters the catheter in your abdomen through a plastic bag. With the catheter sealed, the dialysate remains in your abdomen for four to six hours and is then drained from your abdomen into a bag. Fresh dialysate is then added to start the process over again. You can fold the bag and hide it under your clothes, so no one around you even knows that you're receiving dialysis. With this type of dialysis, you remain in full control of your treatment and can adjust your treatment times to suit your lifestyle. People on CAPD change the dialysate about four times a day.

2. Continuous Cyclic Peritoneal Dialysis (CCPD). Also called automated peritoneal dialysis, this treatment uses a machine called a cycler to exchange the dialysate solution at night: The cycler automatically fills and drains the solution to and from your abdominal cavity, and these treatments take about 10 to 12 hours. Doctors use CCPD to treat people who have problems with CAPD—such as people with hernias or fluid-leak problems. Doctors may also use CCPD for overweight and larger people because they can deliver a higher dose of dialysis this way. Sometimes patients prefer CCPD because they're very busy, and nightly CCPD offers them more free time during the day.

3. Intermittent Peritoneal Dialysis (IPD). Patients treated with IPD undergo dialysis several times a week. (Nightly intermittent peritoneal dialysis, NIPD, is a form of IPD that's particularly attractive.) You may need up to 12 hours of total dialysis time to get enough treatment.

Other helpful advice for patients on peritoneal dialysis:

- Be extra careful about your overall cleanliness and wash your hands frequently to prevent introducing infection into the peritoneal cavity. This infection, called peritonitis, threatens the membrane that is critical to this type of dialysis.

- You may be able to eat more protein. Talk to your doctor for dietary recommendations.

- You may need medications to treat bone disease (vitamin D and phosphate binders), as well as erythropoietin and iron tablets, when you're on peritoneal dialysis.

PERITONEAL DIALYSIS DIAGRAM

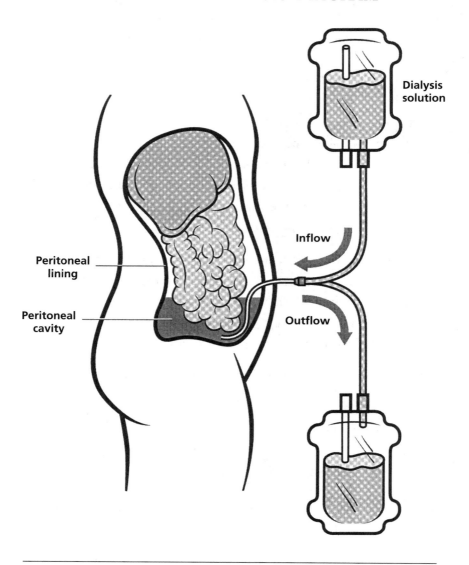

Reprinted with permission from "Getting the Most from Your Treatment: What You Need to Know About Peritoneal Dialysis," ©1998 by the National Kidney Foundation, Inc.

It's important to note that peritoneal dialysis will not affect your sexual function; many men still have normal nature and desire.

KIDNEY TRANSPLANTATION

Transplantation is by far the best treatment for all patients with kidney failure. People who get a kidney transplant live longer and are more likely to live productive lives than people who remain on dialysis. (Sean Elliot, basketball star with the San Antonio Spurs, has received a kidney transplant.) In addition to enhancing the quality of life for ESRD patients, kidney transplantation is less expensive. Nationally, the average medical cost of $16,000 per year for kidney transplantation is much less than the average cost of $46,000 and $41,000 for hemodialysis and peritoneal dialysis, respectively. People can obtain kidneys from living related donors, living unrelated donors, or from cadavers.

Sadly, although 58 percent of people on the waiting list for kidney transplant are black, black people are less likely to agree to donate a kidney for use in transplantation. According to Dr. Clive Callender, chief transplant surgeon at Howard University Hospital, the causes of blacks' reluctance to donate organs include religious beliefs, distrust of the medical establishment, fear of premature death, and racism.[11]

Blacks make up 30 percent of the national kidney waiting list, but obtain only 23 percent of transplanted kidneys. They also wait twice as long for kidneys as whites. Part of the problem is that blacks donate fewer kidneys than whites. A related problem is that there are tissue-typing differences between blacks and whites. Tissue typing—making sure the donor is genetically similar to the recipient—is used to help health officials decide who gets the kidneys that are available. If blacks received more kidneys from fellow blacks, the black recipients would most likely do better. Further, blacks would probably have more opportunity to receive transplants. Efforts are currently underway to increase blacks' awareness of the organ shortage in the United States.

If you're on dialysis and are interested in receiving a kidney transplant, consult your doctor. He or she can advise you on how to begin the process of finding a suitable donor.

CONCLUSION

Proper kidney function is critical for good health. Since the symptoms of kidney disease may not be dramatic in the early phases, it's essential to see your doctor regularly for frequent checkups. And testing is so easy! Simple urine and blood tests can help detect kidney disease early. Proper diet is a key to preventing—and treating—kidney disease.

RESOURCES

American Association of Kidney Patients
100 South Ashley Drive Suite 280
Tampa, FL 33602
(800) 749-2257
(813) 223-0001 (fax)
http://www.aakp.org
(*The Association helps patients locate support groups and offers information and brochures about living a better life as a dialysis patient. The annual membership fee is $25.*)

American Kidney Fund
6110 Executive Boulevard
Suite 1010
Rockville, MD 20852
(800) 638-8299
(301) 881-3052
http://www.akfinc.org
(The Kidney Fund can help you with financial assistance for short-term problems. The organization also offers brochures and pamphlets.)

National Kidney Foundation
30 East 33rd Street, Suite 1100
New York, NY 10016
(800) 622-9010
(212) 889-2210
http://www.kidney.org
(This organization offers brochures and pamphlets on diet, blood pressure, and general kidney disease treatments.)

National Kidney and Urologic Diseases Information Clearinghouse
3 Information Way
Bethesda, MD 20892-3580
(301) 654-4415
(301) 907-8906 (fax)
http://www.niddk.nih.gov/health/urolog/urolog.htm
(The Clearinghouse offers patient education information.)

Polycystic Kidney Research Foundation (PKRF)
4901 Main Street, Suite 200
Kansas City, Missouri 64112-2634
(800) PKD-CURE (800-753-2873)
(816) 931-2600
(816) 931-8655 (fax)
http://www.pkdcure.org/
(PKRF offers patients information about polycystic kidney disease.)

INTERNET RESOURCES

American Society of Nephrology:
http://www.asn-online.com

American Nephrology Nurses' Association:
http://www.annanurse.org

Renal Web:
http://www.renalweb.com

The Complete Website for the Renal Care Community:
http://www.eneph.com

Black Health Online.com:
http://www.blackhealthonline.com

Kidney Directions
http://www.kidneydirections.com
(A website dedicated to discussing kidney disease and transplantation.)

NOTES FOR CHAPTER 8

1. *Southeast Kidney Council, 1996 Annual Report.*
2. Cleveland, W., Marabble, K. G., "Renal failure and donation for transplantation in the African American Community," *Georgia State Medical Association Magazine*, Fall 1999, pp. 19–21.
3. "Incidence and prevalence of ESRD," *USRDS Annual Report 1999*, pp. S40–62.
4. Ibid.
5. Carter, J. S., Pugh, J.A ., Monterrosa, A., "Non-Insulin-Dependent Diabetes Mellitus in Minorities in the United States," *Annals of Internal Medicine*, 1996, vol. 125, pp. 221–232.
6. Guasch, A., Parham, M., Zayas, C. F., Campbell, O., Nzerue, C. M., and Macon, E. "Contrasting Effects of Calcium Channel Blockade versus Converting Enzyme Inhibition on Proteinuria in African Americans with Non-Insulin Dependent Diabetes Mellitus and Nephropathy," *Journal of the American Society of Nephrology*, 1997, vol. 8, pp. 793–798.
7. Carter, J. S., Pugh, J. A., Monterrosa, A., "Non-Insulin-Dependent Diabetes Mellitus in Minorities in the United States," *Annals of Internal Medicine*, 1996, vol. 125, pp. 221–232.
8. "Incidence and prevalence of ESRD," *USRDS Annual Report 1999*, pp. S40–62.
9. Ojo, A. O., Govarts, T. C., Schmoulder, R. L., et al. "Renal Transplantation in End Stage Sickle Cell Nephropathy," *Transplantation*, 1999, vol. 67, pp. 291-295.
10. Ibid.
11. Callender, C. O., Hall, L. E., Yeager, C. L., *New Engl J Med.*, 1991, vol. 325, p. 442.

NINE

AIDS and Sexually Transmitted Diseases

SECTION ONE: AIDS
JASON'S STORY

Even at the advanced stage of his illness, Jason didn't want anyone to know—he even kept his own mother in the dark. She told everyone the same thing he told her: "He just couldn't get rid of his cold, he suspected he was anemic, and, yes, he had lost a great deal of weight, but he was on a terrific new diet." Jason, a young black man in his 20s, has AIDS.

A devoted athlete, Jason always took his body and well-being seriously. Two years ago, he started noticing changes in his health. It seemed as if he was sick with some sort of cold or flu all the time. Each time he got sick, it took him longer to bounce back. Before he started getting sick, Jason ran every morning before work. But about a year ago, he began sleeping in more often, and before long he barely had the energy to get out of bed, let alone put on his shoes and shorts and go running.

During that same period, Jason lost interest in bar-hopping and socializing with his friends. He used to pride himself on being a ladies' man. Several times a week, he'd go to bars and mix and mingle. Sometimes, if he and one of the women he met really hit it off, they would go home together. Jason was very liberal: He saw nothing wrong with casual sex.

What finally convinced him to go to the doctor were the sores that began to appear as small red circles on his legs. That frightened him. It also frightened the last woman he brought home.

Anyone can contract HIV—the virus that causes AIDS—and there are a number of ways to catch the virus. Arthur Ashe, the famous black tennis star, contracted HIV through a blood transfusion. He kept his illness private for years before finally admitting it to the public; then he spent the final 10 months of his life teaching others about the disease before dying in 1993. Ervin "Magic" Johnson, a high-profile basketball player formerly with the Los Angeles Lakers, is also infected with HIV and has gone public with his HIV status to educate people about the disease.

WHAT IS HIV/AIDS?

AIDS (Acquired Immune Deficiency Syndrome) is a disease in which your body's immune system, which normally fends off infections and other diseases, breaks down. When this happens, you are at great risk of contracting life-threatening illnesses such as severe pneumonia, cancer, and nervous system infections. Having AIDS is like being sent to war without armor or ammunition: you're vulnerable to attack and have no way to fight back.

The healthy immune system is constantly fighting many types of viruses. Some viruses, such as those that cause colds, present only minor challenges. Others, such as the human immunodeficiency virus (HIV), can practically destroy your immune system.

As with other viruses, HIV enters your body and immediately begins replicating itself (although studies have shown that HIV can remain inactive in your body for some time before beginning this replication process). Your body may initially put up a strong defense to HIV, and it can take many years before a substantial number of your cells become infected.

Even if you're not yet showing symptoms of HIV, the virus can be detected with blood tests. According to the Centers for Disease Control and Prevention (CDC), 99.8 percent of people infected with HIV will test positive for the virus within six months after infection. By the time you begin to experience AIDS symptoms, your condition may be life threatening.

HOW CAN I PREVENT BECOMING INFECTED WITH HIV?

The best news about HIV/AIDS is that it is preventable. Although it's true that there will be rare accidental HIV infections over which no one has control (for example, a nurse or a doctor may be accidentally stuck with an infected needle), the majority of AIDS cases are caused by unprotected sex or sharing needles when using drugs. You can control these risks. And by taking precautions, you could very well save your own life.

USE CONDOMS

It's the Age of the Condom. Many years ago, condoms were introduced as a birth-control method; today they're also used to protect us from HIV and other sexually transmitted diseases. Not so long ago, it was considered embarrassing to have to go to the drug store to purchase condoms, but today they're handed out on street corners and college campuses and are even sold in their own specialty stores. They're available in every color and style imaginable—even glow-in-the-dark! No matter what color, shape, or design you prefer, be sure to use only condoms made of latex. Latex condoms protect you and your partner from each other's body fluids. The semen of an HIV-infected person will contain the virus, and you want to make it impossible for HIV-infected semen to enter your or your partner's bloodstream.

Just remember: Although condoms are essential in the war against HIV/AIDS, they are *not* 100 percent reliable in protecting you. They may be defective or can break or slip off. Yet as imperfect as condoms may be, they have become essential in fighting the war against HIV/AIDS. The only sure way to avoid the virus is to avoid sharing needles, abstain from sex, or have sex with only one mutually faithful partner who has repeatedly tested negative for HIV.

If you're not sure if you or your partner is infected with HIV, always wear or have your partner wear a condom. You should use a condom for foreplay and afterplay, not just during the sex act itself. You should wear a condom when you put your penis inside the mouth, rectum, or vagina of your partner. You should also use condoms whether your partner is male or female. Protect yourself because no one else is going to do it for you. No one else cares as much as you do—after all, it's *your* life that's at risk.

If you've been tested recently for HIV and the test turned out negative, you're halfway there; now make sure the person you're having sex with is also tested. There's always the chance that even

HOW TO USE A CONDOM

1. PUTTING IT ON

• Use a new condom before each sex act

• When penis is hard (before any sexual contact), place condom on tip and roll down all the way.

• Squeeze tip of condom to remove air. (Excess air could cause condom to break.)

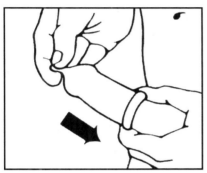

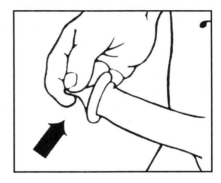

2. TAKING IT OFF

• After coming, withdraw penis while still hard.

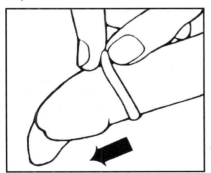

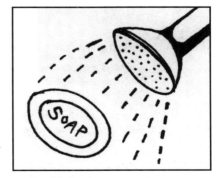

• Hold on to rim of condom as you withdraw so nothing spills.

• Avoid further sexual contact with your partner until both of you wash your sex organs and any other areas that came in contact with body fluids.

though you and your partner have tested negative once, you may be in a "window period"—less than six months after infection—when the virus can't be detected. You must have two tests, six months apart, with no risky behavior in between, in order to be sure you're HIV negative. Unless you're completely sure, always wear a condom, and *never* use a condom more than once.

Condoms are very small and don't take up much room, so make it a practice to carry them with you all the time. Just don't store them in your glove compartment or wallet because heat can destroy the latex. Find a size that's right for you. A loose-fitting condom serves no purpose and will be uncomfortable for you and your partner. Make sure you also check the expiration date because condoms begin to lose their effectiveness after a certain amount of time.

1. Remove the condom from the package carefully, looking for tears in the packaging. Do not open the condom in a way that could rip its latex. (For example, don't use your teeth to rip open the package.) If anything appears at all wrong with the condom, discard it. Risking an unwanted pregnancy or HIV transmission is just not worth it.

2. With your thumb and finger, gently squeeze the tip of the condom. Make sure there will be room in the tip for your semen to collect. Then, place the rolled-up condom at the tip of your erect penis and roll it down to the base of your penis. Prevent any air pockets from forming as you roll it.

3. Lack of lubrication causes problems with condom use; dry friction can cause the condom to tear or break. Water-based lubricants, nonallergenic surgical lubricants (K-Y Jelly), and some contraceptive jellies and foams can be helpful. (Be

sure to read the product labels for use instructions.) These products are available in pharmacies and sex specialty shops. Don't use petroleum jelly or any oil-based lubricant such as hand or body lotion, skin moisturizer, or food products because these will dissolve the condom's latex. Furthermore, don't use saliva, which may contain germs or blood. Try using a contraceptive jelly, cream, or foam that contains nonoxynol-9, which destroys disease-causing germs (including HIV), as it kills sperm.

4. After ejaculation and while it is still erect, remove your penis from your partner's body or have your partner remove his penis. Hold the base of the condom so that its contents do not slip onto your partner. This is important because the penis gets soft after ejaculation, which means the condom may loosen and slip.

5. After use, dispose of the condom carefully so that the semen doesn't spill out. Never reuse a condom or use the same condom for different types of sexual intercourse. New, unused condoms should be used for anal, oral, and vaginal penetration.

DENTAL DAMS

Dental dams are a relatively new concept in safe sex. A dental dam is a square sheet of latex that can be placed over the vagina or anus during oral sex, preventing the exchange of body fluids. (You can purchase dental dams at your local pharmacy.) If you don't have a dental dam, you can unroll a nonlubricated condom and cut it to the right size.

HOW DO I KNOW IF I HAVE HIV?

There's no way to know for sure if you have HIV without having an HIV antibody test. (When the human immunodeficiency virus enters your bloodstream, your immune system produces special antibodies to fight it. This antibody test reveals the presence of HIV antibodies in your blood.)

Some people are reluctant to be tested for HIV because they don't want anyone to know about it if the test turns out to be positive. The solution is to have an anonymous HIV test; no one has to know your name. If you do test positive, however, it's important to consult a health care professional immediately, to talk about the care you'll need. Although researchers haven't yet found a cure for HIV or AIDS, they can often slow the disease's progression and help keep you feeling well for a long time.

TWO TYPES OF HIV TESTS

There are two types of tests used to detect HIV. The first, called ELISA (enzyme-linked immunoabsorbent assay), tests for HIV-related antibodies. This is a very sensitive test, 98 percent accurate, and is the one that the American Red Cross usually uses to test blood that has been donated. Unfortunately, with this test, small particles like proteins and non-HIV antibodies are sometimes mistaken for HIV antibodies and trigger a false positive result. (A "false positive" test result means the test says there's HIV present when it isn't; a "false negative" test result says you're not infected with HIV when you really do have the virus.) To double-check for this mistake, health officials use a second type of test, called "the western blot."

The western blot test is more specific, but it's also more expensive. For this reason, the western blot is used only to confirm a positive ELISA test. An experienced technician, rather than a machine, interprets the results of this test.

BLOOD TEST ACCURACY

If your blood is tested by both the ELISA and the western blot tests, you can be fairly sure that the results are accurate. In rare instances, false positives and false negatives have been reported. False negatives occur most often during the "window" period, which is the period of time after you've been infected with HIV, but before your body has built up enough HIV antibodies to be detected by an ELISA test. If you know that you've been exposed to HIV, get tested at regular intervals so that you can be sure of getting an accurate result.

Test results, depending on which kind of test is used and where you're tested, usually take about a week to get back. If you have a high risk of being exposed to HIV, even if your initial test was negative, you should have a follow-up test six weeks and six months after the suspected exposure. And make sure you avoid unsafe sex and drug use during this period of time, and always.

WHERE SHOULD I GET TESTED?

You can have an HIV antibody test at most clinics, local health departments, hospitals, or doctors' offices. However, if you are tested at any one of these places, there's no guarantee that your results will be kept confidential. Some hospitals and doctors are required by law to report those people who test positive for HIV. If you want to be assured of confidentiality, go to a site that offers anonymous testing. Call the Centers for Disease Control National AIDS Hotline (800-342-AIDS) for information on anonymous testing sites in your area, or call your state health department. Many state and county health departments provide these blood tests free of charge for people who can't afford the fee.

TREATMENT

Imagine yourself in this situation: You decide to have an HIV test. After all, you may have done something in your past, before AIDS became a threat that put you at risk. Days later, the results come back. You have tested positive for being infected with HIV. Now what? Fear, anger, frustration, helplessness—you may feel all these natural reactions. You've seen movies and read stories about people with AIDS. But this time, it's you.

Don't lose hope! Research is going on every day to find a cure for this disease. Prescription medicines can help prevent and treat HIV-related infections, and many of them can slow down the virus as it attacks your immune system. New drugs are being tested all over the world; clinical drug trials can give you access to these investigational therapies.

THE STAGES OF HIV

Remember that a positive test for HIV doesn't necessarily mean you have AIDS; it means you have HIV. If you're infected with HIV, it's important to understand the changes that your body is going through.

1. *Before HIV antibodies show up on a test:* You can be infected with HIV but not have enough antibodies to be detected by a test. This window period, which we mentioned earlier, can last for several weeks or months after infection.

2. *HIV positive, but showing no symptoms:* If you've been told that you're HIV positive, or if you suspect that you have been exposed to HIV but have no symptoms, you may be particularly dangerous to others. Because you may not be aware of your illness, you may continue practicing unsafe sex or other risky behaviors. Your sex or needle-sharing partner(s) may also be less likely to take precautions since you don't appear to be ill.

3. *HIV positive, showing symptoms:* If you've been told that you have HIV and have begun showing signs or symptoms, such as swollen glands, weight loss, diarrhea, or skin rashes, you're at this stage. Your physical condition may gradually worsen, and you may find it necessary to alter your daily activities.

4. *Acquired Immune Deficiency Syndrome (AIDS):* This is the full-blown phase of the HIV infection. This is when you're most prone to opportunistic infections and certain cancers. Illnesses that you may experience are recurrent lung infections, anemia (decreased red blood cells), more severe skin conditions such as Kaposi's sarcoma (a form of cancer), kidney dysfunction, dementia, and drastic weight loss. Nerve damage can also result in blindness, loss of hearing, and walking difficulties.

JASON FACES THE TRUTH

Jason decided to go to a health clinic to have his blood tested for HIV. A nurse took his blood and gave him some pamphlets to read. A doctor came in and advised him to abstain from sex while he was wait-

*ing for his test results. That was okay with him; he didn't really feel
all that well anyway.*

*After a week, Jason got his test results. He had tested positive for
HIV. Although the appearance of the sores on his body had hinted
at a serious illness, Jason never thought he had AIDS. After all, he
wasn't gay and he didn't do drugs.*

*Jason went back to the clinic to see if they could have made a
mistake. The doctor there said that they could test him again
because false-positive test results have occurred before; however, the
sores on Jason's legs looked suspiciously like Kaposi's sarcoma, a skin
condition often seen among AIDS patients. Jason took another test.
While awaiting his second set of test results, he suffered silently,
afraid to say anything to friends, ex-girlfriends, or his family. The
second test results, too, came back positive for HIV.*

*Jason immediately met with the clinic doctor, who advised him
to tell all of his former or present sex partners of the blood test
results. Jason says it was the hardest thing he's ever had to do in his
life. Some of his previous partners, knowing that Jason had infected
them only because he was unaware of his disease, took it well.
Others cried or yelled at him, blaming him for putting them at risk.
It was no use arguing with them that they had put themselves at risk
as well. Jason was overcome with guilt and sincerely hoped that
none of his former sex partners tested positive.*

AIDS IN THE BLACK POPULATION

Among black men 25 to 44 years old, HIV infection has been the
leading cause of death since 1991, when it surpassed homicide in
the ranking of causes of death. HIV infection caused nearly 9,000
deaths, or 32 percent of all deaths in this group at its peak in

1995. In 1998, the infection caused 3,000 deaths, or 16 percent of the total. Overall, in the United States the incidence of HIV infection peaked approximately 15 years ago, and the annual number of HIV infections has been stable at approximately 40,000 since 1992. When the CDC estimated the prevalence of HIV infection at the end of 1998, it was in the range of 800,000 to 900,000 infected people. Of these people, approximately 625,000 had had HIV infection or had been diagnosed with AIDS (CDC, unpublished data, 1999).

According to estimates from the Joint United Nations Programme on HIV/AIDS (UNAIDS) and the World Health Organization (WHO), 32.2 million adults and 1.2 million children will be living with HIV by the end of 1999.[1]

According to CDC estimates, there were approximately 118,525 black people living with AIDS in 1998, and approximately 8,401 blacks died from the disease in that year.[2] In 1998, 62 percent of women[3] and children with AIDS were black.[4]

The CDC also reports that as of June 1999, 711,344 cases of AIDS were documented in the United States.[5] Of that number, 192,092 AIDS patient were black men over 13 years old. White males with AIDS totaled 284,484; Hispanics, 104,628; Asian Americans, 4,499.[6]

In the early 1980s, AIDS was viewed as a disease of gay white men. But according to the CDC, the proportional distribution of AIDS cases among racial–ethnic groups has shifted since 1985: The proportion of cases among whites has decreased over time, while cases among blacks and Hispanics have increased.[7]

"We had an epidemic on our hands," Sandra McDonald says. McDonald is the president and founder of Outreach, Inc., a support service for people with AIDS in Atlanta, Georgia. McDonald

AIDS CASES BY AGE AND SEX:
REPORTED 1981-1998

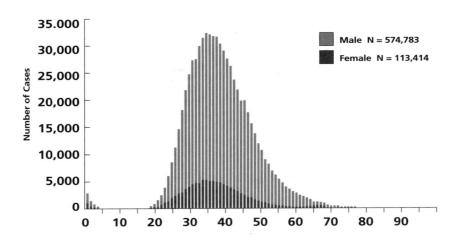

Reprinted from Centers for Disease Control and Prevention, Divisions of HIV/AIDS Website.

lowered her voice. "In the New Jersey and New York areas, hundreds of young black men were dying and everyone assumed it was from drug overdoses. In 1989, 100 bodies were exhumed. Guess what? Many of them had AIDS. By then, our black communities had already been infected and affected for a long time."

Outreach, Inc. opened its doors in 1986. McDonald ministered to the gay white community for six months before she helped her first black gay man in July 1986. "I couldn't find one," she said. "Because of the stigma attached to being gay in the black community, many homosexuals preferred being classified as intravenous (IV) drug users rather than gay."

McDonald said, "There has always been homosexuality in the African American community, but we never talked about it. Why?

We were aware of it, but we didn't embrace it. If we don't embrace something, we can't empower it. So, instead, we have chosen to ignore homosexuality."

Sedrick Gardner, director of programs for Outreach, Inc., has worked full time with McDonald for three years. "We are here to help everyone," said Gardner. "AIDS can be absolutely devastating. But with society the way it is, it may very well be most difficult for a black and gay patient to deal with AIDS.

"As a black man, the gay must deal with racism every day. If he is out of the closet, in many cases he must learn to live without the support of his family, so he must rely on the support of close friends if he has them. If he is open about his homosexuality in his personal life, but not with his co-workers, he may constantly live with the fear that someone at work will find out. If he has chosen to live the 'straight life,' then he may be hounded continually by the universal aunt who can't understand why he isn't married yet.

"When this man comes home from work, he must remove masks and peel back layers of his persona to find himself. He has to suffer all of this because society has chosen to judge him strictly by a sex act, and not as a whole person. So many black men are dying from high blood pressure, heart disease, stress, homicide, and now AIDS. We've lost one generation to war, drugs, and crime. We're about to lose another to AIDS."

Historically, ministers in black churches would not discuss any type of sexuality—it was a taboo subject. But national efforts by Rev. Joseph E. Lowery, president of the Southern Christian Leadership Conference, and especially his declaration that AIDS is a "civil rights issue" for blacks, have encouraged other ministers to become more involved. In fact, many large black churches have had AIDS ministries since the late 1980s. The work of these min-

AIDS RATES PER 100,000 BLACK POPULATION: REPORTED IN 1998

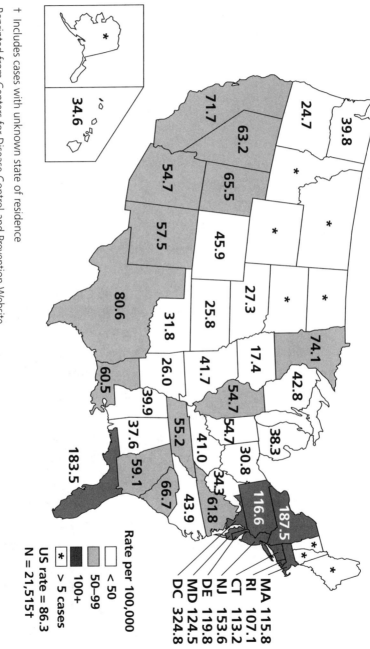

† Includes cases with unknown state of residence
Reprinted from Centers for Disease Control and Prevention Website.

34.6

*

39.8
24.7
71.7
63.2
65.5
54.7
57.5
45.9
27.3
*
*
*
80.6
31.8
25.8
41.7
17.4
*
74.1
42.8
26.0
39.9
54.7
54.7
38.3
60.5
37.6
55.2
41.0
30.8
34.3
61.8
183.5
59.1
66.7
43.9
116.6
187.5
*
*
*

Rate per 100,000
< 50
50–99
100+
* > 5 cases
US rate = 86.3
N = 21,515†

MA 115.8
RI 107.1
CT 113.2
NJ 153.6
DE 119.8
MD 124.5
DC 324.8

istries includes providing meals daily for people with AIDS, implementing buddy programs to provide emotional support, and establishing housing programs.

John Templeton, director of AIDS education at Grady Memorial Hospital in Atlanta, shared a frightening statistic: "When I came here five years ago, the AIDS clinic at the hospital was located in a small, dark corner, and patients had to wait two or three weeks for an appointment. Now we are in a big, new building, on two floors, and patients must still wait a long time for an appointment."

McDonald and others insist that things are getting better in the black community for gays and IV drug users. Those who cross the threshold of Outreach, Inc., receive warmth, love, and acceptance. They also receive education, pamphlets, and counseling. "There is no cure," said McDonald. "The only weapon we have to fight AIDS with is education."

JASON INVESTIGATES THE CAUSE OF HIS HIV INFECTION

Jason found it very difficult to tell his past sexual partners he had been diagnosed with HIV. During one such conversation, an old girlfriend confided that she, too, had been diagnosed with HIV several years before. Perhaps he had gotten the AIDS virus from unprotected sex with her. He would probably never know. What he did know was that when he was sleeping with her he did not use condoms regularly. Sure, if either of them had had a condom at the time, he would have put it on. But sometimes he forgot to bring one, and it never occurred to either of them to put their passion on hold while Jason went out to buy a condom. Now Jason wished that he had.

AM I AT RISK?

Anyone can get AIDS. Period. You don't have to be a male homosexual to contract HIV. In fact, the number of documented cases of
AIDS in homosexuals is decreasing annually, whereas the number
of heterosexuals testing positive for HIV is rising steadily. By simply
letting your guard down one time, you can get this fatal disease.

"AIDS is a serious epidemic," says Templeton. "Anyone who
has shared needles or who has been sexually active during the last
10 years needs an HIV test. There are ways for those who are HIV
positive to improve the quality of their lives. But before they can
seek help, they need to know if they are infected."

CDC documentation indicates that HIV has been in the
United States since at least 1978. Although homosexual men were
historically the first group associated with AIDS, the heterosexual
community is quickly catching up. The CDC has compiled a list
of questions to help you determine if you're at risk of becoming
infected with HIV. If any of the following known risk factors
apply to you, consider being tested:

- If you are a male, have you had sex with other males?

- Have you shared needles or syringes to inject drugs?

- Have you had sex with someone who may have been
  infected with HIV?

- Have you had a sexually transmitted disease?

- Did you receive blood transfusions or blood products
  between 1978 and 1985?

- Have you had sex with someone who could answer yes to
  any of the preceding questions?

- Have you had unprotected sex with someone whose HIV status you do not know?

HOW CAN I BECOME INFECTED BY HIV?

In order for HIV to be passed from another person to you, the virus must be carried from inside the infected person's body to the inside of your body, and then to your bloodstream. This can happen through an open wound or one of your many body openings. Often, the virus will first enter through one of your mucous membranes, and then pass to your nearby blood vessels.

HIV can be transmitted by a variety of fluids to your body, such as blood, semen, secretions from the vagina and cervix, and breast milk. In some HIV-infected individuals, traces of the virus have been found in tears, urine, saliva, and feces, but in insufficient quantities to transmit the infection to another person. Feces and urine pose a risk only if blood is present. HIV is most concentrated in semen, blood, and vaginal and cervical secretions.

BLOOD TRANSMISSION

Have you noticed that your dentist now wears rubber gloves, goggles or glasses, and a surgical mask while he or she works on your teeth? Have you noticed that a professional or college basketball game stops if a player gets injured and starts bleeding? The player then has to change the part of the uniform that has blood on it, the blood must be wiped up from the floor, and the floor is cleaned with a disinfectant. This procedure may seem overly cautious, but people are becoming aware of the dangers of getting HIV through blood.

The bottom line: It's dangerous to come in contact with someone else's blood. You have no idea whether or not that person is infected with HIV or other germs that may be transmitted through blood. We often have openings on our skin in the form of tiny cuts and splits, most commonly around our fingernails. Blood can, although very rarely, enter these openings, carrying HIV with it. The chances are remote, but it is possible to become infected in this way.

Some infected drug users don't care whether or not the needles they use are clean, so now many of them are either infected with HIV or have AIDS. If one drug user out of five has HIV and shares the needle with his or her other four friends, he or she is thoughtlessly spreading the virus at a rapid pace.

At one time, having a blood transfusion or organ transplant was risky. Because HIV wasn't discovered until 1983, neither blood nor organ donors were tested for the disease. As a result, some people who required blood transfusions in the late 1970s and early 1980s acquired the disease through the blood of donors with AIDS. Arthur Ashe, for example, acquired HIV from a blood transfusion during heart surgery. Similarly, some people who had been given a second chance to live through an organ donation were unfortunately infected with HIV as a result.

Today, the chance of getting HIV through a blood transfusion is remote. Since 1985, screening of blood and organs for HIV has become very strict, and donating blood is safe. New needles are used for each donor, and all blood is tested for HIV before it's used. Even so, you shouldn't donate blood if you're at high risk of having HIV. If you want to know if you have HIV, get tested at a clinic or by a doctor. *Do not donate blood in order to be tested for the virus.*

EXPOSURE TO SEMEN

Semen ejaculates from your penis during orgasm. A person with an HIV infection may have a high concentration of HIV in this fluid. HIV can also be found in the pre-ejaculatory fluid that comes from the tip of the penis. During unprotected vaginal intercourse, HIV from the semen can go across the mucous membrane of the vagina or cervix and can travel through the membrane to tiny blood vessels found nearby. Any abrasions or breaks in the membrane make transmission of the virus even more likely. During vaginal intercourse, the woman (the receptor) is the one most at risk.

Anal intercourse seems to be the most risky form of sex when it comes to getting HIV. As in the vagina, there is a mucous membrane in the rectum that can serve as a passageway, enabling the highly concentrated HIV found in semen to travel to the receptor's bloodstream. The rectum is designed less well than the vagina to block passage of the virus. Further, the rectum tends to have more small tears than the vaginal membrane. During anal intercourse, the receptor, whether male or female, is the one most at risk.

HIV may also be transmitted through oral sex since the mouth is lined with mucous membranes, too. If you have breaks or small cuts in the skin of your mouth, your risk of contracting the virus from an oral sex partner increases. During vaginal, anal, and oral intercourse, using a condom or dental dam will help prevent you or your partner from acquiring HIV.

CONTACT WITH VAGINAL AND
CERVICAL SECRETIONS

Secretions from the vagina and cervix can carry HIV although concentrations of the virus generally aren't as high as in semen

and blood. Using a condom is important because it can help protect the male from getting HIV from the female, as well as protect
the female from getting HIV and other sexually transmitted diseases from the male.

PREGNANCY

There is an approximately 25 to 30 percent chance that a pregnant woman with HIV can pass the virus to her unborn child
through her blood or through breastfeeding after the baby is
born. HIV-positive women should discuss with a doctor the risk
of passing their infection on to a baby.

WAYS YOU CANNOT GET HIV

It's important to know how you can't get HIV. You can't become
infected from:

- Sitting on a toilet seat
- Eating food prepared by someone who has the virus
- Holding, hugging, or touching a person who has the virus
- Swimming in a pool with someone who has the virus
- Working with or attending school with someone who has
  the virus
- Being bitten by a mosquito

Although a very small amount of HIV has been found in
tears, saliva, urine, and feces, there have been no documented
cases of anyone getting the disease from these materials because
the concentration of HIV in them is too low.

WHAT COMPLICATIONS CAN I DEVELOP IF I HAVE AIDS?

AIDS can affect virtually every part of your body. Changes in your skin, major organs, weight, and energy level are the most obvious examples. The complications you experience will be, for the most part, a result of your immune system getting weaker, opening the door to other diseases.

Your Immune System Will Be Affected

Your body's immune system is made up of a variety of organs and cells that work to rid your body of foreign substances, such as bacteria and viruses. Some of the white blood cells in your immune system, known as CD4, T cells, T4 cells, or helper lymphocytes (all different names for the same cell), normally assist your immune system in fighting disease. If you have HIV, these cells are killed for reasons not completely understood.

If you don't have HIV, your CD4 cell level is usually above 500 cells per cubic millimeters of blood. (This number indicates the amount of CD4 cells in your body.) For the AIDS patient, this number usually declines as the virus gains a foothold. As of 1993, you are considered to have AIDS by the medical community when your CD4 level dips below 200. Once this happens, you may be put on preventive medicines such as Bactrim, which can help prevent infections that your immune system can no longer fight. You may also be offered one or more drugs that act directly on the HIV to reduce its impact on your body. These drugs go by the strange acronyms of AZT, ddl, ddC, and + d_4T. If you're HIV positive, your CD4 count should be monitored every four to six months.

Some germs will take advantage of a low CD4 cell concentration or weakened immune system, and cause infections and disease. These include a variety of fungal, parasitic, and viral infections and certain unusual bacterial infections, such as tuberculosis (TB). In fact, TB is becoming a major problem among people who are infected with HIV.

You May Develop Skin Disorders

Sometimes patients with AIDS (Jason, for example) will develop skin disorders, such as Kaposi's sarcoma, a rare cancer. Kaposi's sarcoma can appear in all shapes, sizes, and colors on your skin though it usually appears as bruising or blotching. It can also appear anywhere inside or outside your body. Other types of skin disorders that are prevalent among AIDS patients include herpes (a viral infection, which presents itself as blisters) and psoriasis (skin lesions that appear as thickened red areas covered by white scales on your skin). Another common skin problem among HIV patients is a rash that appears on your scalp, face, and neck.

You May Develop a Pneumocystis Carinii Pneumonia (PCP) Infection

PCP, a lung disorder caused by a special class of bacteria, was rare before the AIDS epidemic. If you have HIV, the PCP infection can more easily cause disease because of your weakened immune system. Symptoms of PCP are shortness of breath, a cough, and fever. Approximately 60 to 80 percent of all AIDS patients contract this disorder. A variety of medications are available to treat this type of pneumonia and prevent it.

You May Lose Weight

One of the symptoms of HIV infection is progressive weight loss. The human immunodeficiency virus can cause your body to burn energy at a higher rate than normal. If you're HIV positive, you'll need to increase your calorie intake and use vitamin supplements to keep up with the drastic changes your body is experiencing. (Not all HIV-positive people have this problem.)

Other HIV-related factors that have to do with weight loss are diarrhea and malnutrition. Diarrhea can be a side effect of prescription medication, a sign of serious infection, or simply a symptom of HIV. Whatever the source, if you have diarrhea for more than a few days, you should notify your doctor. Diarrhea can cause dehydration, which can lead to other serious health problems. In severe cases of diarrhea, you may experience malnutrition because your food passes through your digestive system too quickly for nutrients to be properly absorbed.

Your Kidneys May Fail

HIV/AIDS can also cause your kidneys to malfunction. Because HIV breaks down your body's immune system, every other body system can be affected. If your kidneys become infected, a variety of life-threatening disorders can occur. Read Chapter 8 for more specific information about kidney failure.

You May Lose Your Sight

Because of nerve damage caused by HIV-related infections (specifically, an opportunistic virus called CMV), you can lose your sight to this disease. Some opportunistic infections may take advantage of your weakened system and cause a condition called retinitis, which can lead to blindness. If this disease is caught early enough, it can be treated.

JASON TAKES CHARGE OF HIS FATE

Once Jason was certain he had AIDS, he could only go through the motions of his everyday life. He went to work, came home, and kept to himself. He was feeling sorry for himself and didn't want others to watch. One day a co-worker friend asked Jason if he was feeling all right. The co-worker could tell that Jason had lost a lot of weight, and knew that he had used several of his sick days. Jason, tired of the solitude, confided in his friend, telling him of his diagnosis. "What are you doing about it?" the co-worker asked. The question caught Jason off guard. After all, everyone knows there's no cure for AIDS. "Nothing," Jason responded with a shrug.

The next day, his friend approached him with an armful of pamphlets, magazine articles, and library books concerning the treatment of HIV/AIDS. After work, the two men pored over all the information, learning about the various forms of treatments. Today, Jason takes several prescription drugs to help control the complications of HIV, and he is also waiting to be called to participate in a clinical trial.

YOU CAN PARTICIPATE IN A CLINICAL TRIAL

A clinical trial is a test of a new drug on people with HIV. When a research laboratory develops a new drug for AIDS patients, there's no way to know how the drug will work or what the side effects will be. First, the drug is tested in a test tube in the laboratory, then on animals. After that, the researchers need human volunteers. Since there's no cure for AIDS or HIV, many volunteers feel as though they have nothing to lose by trying an experimental drug. (Some of these investigational drugs have been very helpful for people who participated in these trials.) Before participating in a drug trial, you'll be given lots of information about the potential risks and benefits of the drug you will be taking. Researchers will screen you carefully before they allow you to participate.

Remember, if you decide to participate, there's no guarantee of recovery. The drug or treatment being test may not work at all, or may even make your condition worse. You have to decide if it's worth the risk to you. Be assured that you can leave the trial and stop taking the treatment at any time. To find out more about clinical trials, see the information located at the end of this chapter. Unfortunately, many trials are very limited and can accommodate only a small fraction of the number of people who are interested.

AIDS SUPPORT

If you're infected with HIV, support is essential. It's hard enough to cope with the disease, much less cope with it alone. Many hotline services, outreach programs, and support systems are available to lend you support.

Sandra McDonald's Outreach, Inc., is one example. "We don't point fingers here," said McDonald. "Everyone who walks through our door is a family member." Located on the southwest side of Atlanta, Outreach, Inc., exemplifies grassroots programs located in major cities throughout the country.

"People I had known all my life avoided me when I started this organization," McDonald said. "For years I rented space in downtown Atlanta because I couldn't get space in this part of town. Those damn bastards thought they would get the disease."

Sedrick Gardner facilitates several workshops at Outreach, Inc. for black men who are HIV positive. "I've seen life just turn around for some of these men," he said. "In a group, they learn to help themselves and each other. They come from all walks of life—lawyers, teachers, accountants, musicians and clerks. If you ran into the group on the street, you would never think it was an HIV support group. I've learned a lot from these men. AIDS is about life. It is not about death. Men suffering with this disease know what is important and live each day to the fullest. All of us could learn something from them."

If you'd like information about services like Outreach, Inc., which are available throughout the country, call the AIDS Hotline given at the end of this chapter. The person who answers your call will be happy to provide you with the information you need.

SECTION TWO:
SEXUALLY TRANSMITTED DISEASES
Billy Has a Dilemma

Billy was 18 years old and had been sexually active for the past three years. He was crazy about his new girlfriend, Kellie, and knew that he was the first boy with whom she had ever been intimate. How was he going to explain to Kellie and to his parents that he had probably given Kellie gonorrhea and that she needed to be examined right away?

OTHER SEXUALLY TRANSMITTED DISEASES

If you have been diagnosed with a sexually transmitted disease (STD), you should tell your partners. All of them. There are many sexually transmitted diseases in addition to HIV infection of which you should be aware. Like HIV, these infections spread from one person to another during sexual contact.

According to *Healthy People 2010: National Health Promotion and Disease Prevention Objectives*, STD refers to more than 25 infectious organisms that are primarily transmitted through sexual activity.[8] Although most of these diseases have been known for a long time, new diagnostic methods have helped investigators describe how widespread they are, how they're transmitted, and what their consequences are. Almost 15 million cases of STD occur annually in the United States, including 4 million cases among teenagers.[9] By age 21, approximately one out of every five young Americans requires treatment for a sexually transmitted disease. The total societal cost of sexually transmitted diseases, including sexually transmitted HIV infection, exceeds $17 billion annually.[10]

Anyone can contract a sexually transmitted disease—whether rich, poor, young, old, black, or white. And if you have sexual contact with anyone with an STD, you can catch it.

GONORRHEA

Gonorrhea is a treatable localized infection involving your genitals and urinary tract. If you have contact with an infected person, you may experience gonorrhea symptoms on the same day or within 1 to 14 days. (The majority of men develop symptoms within two to five days.) Your symptoms may include genital discharge and burning when you urinate. These symptoms are more easily recognized by men, but often go unnoticed by both men and women. Since 1990, gonorrhea rates have decreased for all racial and ethnic groups. However, large racial and ethnic disparities still exist, especially among young people.[11]

A major barrier to further reducing the incidence of gonorrhea is an increase in antibiotic-resistant strains. In 1996, 29 percent of gonorrhea organisms were resistant to penicillin, tetracycline, or both.[12] If antibiotics don't cure gonorrhea or if the infection is antibiotic resistant, it can cause sterility, arthritis, blindness, or damage to your urinary tract. If a pregnant woman has gonorrhea, it can also cause blindness in her unborn child.[13]

SYPHILIS

Syphilis affects your entire body system and has the potential to do even more damage than gonorrhea. There are three stages in the development of syphilis. In the primary stage, a painless sore or chancre appears at the place where the germ first entered your body (usually around the genitals). The time between picking up the germ via sexual contact with an infected person and the appearance of the first symptom can range from 10 to 90 days (the average is 21 days). The chancre can go unnoticed, especially in women, and will disappear on its own with or without treatment, as the disease goes into the next stage.

The secondary stage of syphilis is characterized by skin rashes, hair loss, sore throat, fever, and headaches. These symptoms may last two to six weeks (four weeks average) and disappear on their own without treatment. In the final stage, the disease goes deeper into your body until it reappears years later after doing irreparable damage. Untreated, syphilis can cause blindness, deafness, heart disease, insanity, and eventually, death. Women who have the disease when they are pregnant may give

birth to children who are handicapped or stillborn. As with gonorrhea, doctors can treat syphilis with antibiotics. It is easiest to
treat in the first and second stage.

HERPES SIMPLEX

Herpes simplex is a virus that affects your genito-urinary system.
Symptoms appear from 2 to 20 days after you've had contact with
an infected partner. You may experience one or groups of small
bumps or blisters in your genital area—on, around, or inside the
vagina; on the penis; or in or around the anus. These blisters can
be very painful and uncomfortable, and you may also feel ill. The
blisters usually begin to dry up and disappear within 5 to 20 days.

There's no cure for herpes, but there is treatment. You can
infect another person anytime, even when your symptoms aren't
acting up. When the blisters disappear, the virus remains in your
body, and symptoms may recur when you're tired or run down,
or when you have a cold, fever, or sunburn. Emotional upsets and
stress may also bring on a recurrence. Drugs can ease the symptoms, decrease the duration of the attack, and help prevent recur-
rences. But, again, there is no cure for herpes.

VENEREAL WARTS

Venereal warts are also caused by a virus; symptoms usually
develop 30 to 90 days after you have had contact with an infected
partner. These small warts can appear anywhere in and around
the penis, vagina, or anus. They don't usually hurt or itch, and
may go unnoticed unless you look for them or discover them by
touch.

As long as you have symptoms, you're contagious. Even after the warts disappear, the virus remains in your body, and may recur when you're tired and run down. Although there's no cure for venereal warts, they can be managed if they're frozen or burned off.

CHLAMYDIA

Of all the infectious diseases mentioned here, chlamydia is probably the least known among the general population, yet paradoxically, it is the most frequent sexually transmitted germ in the United States. *Healthy People 2010* researchers estimate that 4 million acute infections occur annually from this organism. Many people with the disease have no symptoms or signs of infection. Inflammation of the male urethra, the duct that transports urine from the bladder through the prostate and penis is called urethritis, and 35 to 50 percent of these infections are caused by the chlamydia microorganism. Thanks to recent research advances, accurate urine tests are now available. These new tests make testing of males more feasible and less uncomfortable than other chlamydia tests. Additionally, single-dose antibiotic therapy promises to substantially enhance the likelihood of successful treatment—especially in adolescents—as compared to the commonly used seven-day oral medication.[14]

OTHER INFECTIONS

There are some common vaginal infections that women can contract and pass on to a partner. These include bacterial infections, yeast infections, or trichomonas infections. Some of the symptoms of these infections include discharge, itching, a foul odor, painful or frequent urination, and dryness and sensitivity around and inside the vagina. In addition, men often get infections that produce discharge, painful or frequent urination, and penile sensitivity. These infections can also be passed on to a partner.

PUBIC LICE AND SCABIES

Pubic lice, commonly called crabs, are animals about the size of a pinhead that live in the hairy areas of your genitals and other hairy parts of your body. Some people experience intense itching or rashes, whereas others, who are not allergic to the lice bite, may not experience symptoms. You can cure crabs by applying a specially prescribed medicated soap or shampoo.

Scabies are mites that leave small, raised reddish tracts on your skin. Scabies cause your skin to itch and can be transmitted venereally through close body contact. They're highly infectious. Your doctor can prescribe a number of different creams or lotions to cure scabies.

A SPECIAL NOTE ABOUT TUBERCULOSIS

Tuberculosis is not considered a "sexually transmitted disease" because it is airborne. Moreover, it was in decline for decades. From 1953 to 1985, the number of TB cases reported annually in the United States dropped 74 percent, from 84,304 to 22,201. Physicians and medical professionals were congratulating each other on the supposed elimination of tuberculosis (TB) in the United States.

However, this trend stopped between 1985 and 1992, when there was a 20 percent increase in the number of persons reported with TB, several of whom were diagnosed with multidrug-resistant strains of Mycobacterium tuberculosis, which causes TB. As a result, health agencies needed to respond to the new TB threat: They used their resources to ensure that all people with TB were promptly diagnosed and were tested for drug resistance. Most of these people were offered therapy and referrals to other necessary health and social services.

As a result of this quick action, TB cases have decreased by 34 percent from 1992 through 1999 (the last year for which there is available information). Additionally, the percent of multidrug-resistant TB strains has declined from almost 3 percent in 1993 to 1.1 percent in 1998. However, although multidrug-resistant TB cases were reported from 19 states in 1993, by 1998, they were reported from 45 states, making it necessary for all health departments to be prepared to address the unique problems posed by persons with this form of TB.

Despite the recent declines, TB remains an important problem in people with HIV infection, in people who are potentially exposed to others with TB in congregate settings (such as prisons, jails, and homeless shelters), and in foreign-born people—reflecting the global magnitude of TB's menace. The World Health Organization has estimated that approximately one-third of the world's population is infected with Mycobacterium tuberculosis, about 8 million people are diagnosed with TB, and 2 million die of TB every year. Another 1 million people with HIV/AIDS die of TB, making TB the leading infectious killer of the world. Current efforts are underway to improve the ability to mount a global fight against TB.

Public health agencies need to target people at risk for TB infection to make sure they're screened with the tuberculin skin test. If the test comes back positive, these agencies should offer (a highly effective) treatment for latent TB infection called preventive therapy. Different treatment options are now recommended by the American Thoracic Society and the Centers for Disease Control and Prevention.

If you suffer from a persistent cough, weight loss, or night sweats, you should be evaluated by a medical professional to rule out TB. People who are diagnosed with TB should be treated, preferably under direct observation, to make sure that they complete a full course of anti-TB therapy with multiple drugs. Any people with whom they've had contact must also be evaluated for the possibility of TB disease or latent TB infection.

CONCLUSION

The important thing to remember about AIDS and other STDs is that you can avoid virtually every disease and infection (except perhaps tuberculosis) mentioned in this chapter. The best way to avoid becoming infected with HIV (the virus that causes AIDS), as well as other sexually transmitted diseases is by avoiding the high-risk behaviors listed in this chapter. Although condoms alone do not provide complete protection, they do reduce your chances of becoming infected with HIV or other sexually transmitted infections.

Use latex condoms properly every time you have sex—vaginal, anal, or oral. You can also prevent an HIV infection by abstaining from sex completely or by having sex with only one mutually faithful, uninfected partner, and by not sharing needles. Know that if you take precautions sexually transmitted infections do not have to be a part of your life.

If you suspect you've been exposed to someone infected with an STD, keep in mind that these infections are very common and are nothing to be embarrassed about. See a medical professional immediately because early treatment can help to prevent long-term damage. Continue to follow the guidelines in this chapter to ensure that you're getting the best care possible and preventing others from becoming infected. Remember, you're the most important part of your own health care plan.

RESOURCES

CDC National Prevention Information Network (NPIN)
P.O. Box 6003
Rockville, MD 20849-6003
(800) 458-5231
(301) 562-1098
(301) 562-1098 (international)
(301) 588-1589 (international TTY)
(800) 243-7012 (TTY)
info@cdcnpin.org (e-mail address)
(National reference, referral, and distribution service for information on HIV/AIDS, STDs, and TB, sponsored by the Centers for Disease Control and Prevention.)

American Red Cross
431 18th Street
Washington, DC 20006
(202) 639-3520
http://www.redcross.org
(Contact your local chapter for resources, programs, brochures on AIDS, training classes, and services.)

Centers for Disease Control and Prevention (CDC)
1600 Clifton Road, N.E.
Atlanta, GA 30333
(888) 232-3228
http://www.cdc.gov
(This organization provides information through telephone voice messages, fax machines, or the mail.)

The Department of Public Health
(Contact your local or state department of public health for HIV and AIDS information.)

National AIDS Hotline
(800) 342-2437
(800) 342-AIDS
(800) 243-7889 (for persons with hearing impairments)
(When you call the hotline, staff members will answer your questions regarding AIDS. They will also send brochures when requested and make referrals.)

SIDA National AIDS Hotline (Spanish)
(800) 344-7432
(800) 344-SIDA
(When you call the hotline, staff members will answer your questions regarding AIDS. They will also send brochures when requested and make referrals.)

National Association of People With AIDS
1413 K Street N. W.
Washington, DC 20005
(202) 898-0414
(202) 898-0435 (fax)
(This group provides supportive services to AIDS patients and will put you in touch with local chapters when you call.)

National Institute of Allergy and Infectious Diseases (NIAID)
AIDS Clinical Trials Information Service
P.O. Box 6421
Rockville, MD 20849-6421
(800) 874-2572
(800) TRIALS-A
(This service offers clinical trial information.)

The Rotary Club
(The Rotary Club in Los Altos, California, has produced an educational videotape about HIV and AIDS called "The Los Altos Story." Contact your local Rotary Club for information on obtaining the tape.)

National STD Hotline
(800) 227-8922

National Herpes Hotline
(919) 361-8488

National Prevention Information Network
(800) 458-5231

American Social Health Association

P.O. Box 13827

Research Triangle Park, NC 27709

(919) 361-8400

(919) 361-8425 Fax

http://www.ashastd.org

(The Association offers educational, patient advocacy, and support group services.)

State Agencies

(Look up AIDS under "state agencies" in your local phone book to find out about financial aid programs.)

NOTES FOR CHAPTER 9

1. Joint United Nations Programme on HIV/AIDS (UNAIDS) and the World Health Organization (WHO), December 1999. Source: http://www.unaids.org/hivaidsinfo/documents.html
2. Centers for Disease Control and Prevention, *HIV/AIDS Surveillance Report, 1999*; 11 (No.1): pp. 34, 36. Source: http://www.cdc.gov/nchstp/hiv_aids/stats/hasrlink.htm
3. CDC HIV/AIDS Surveillance in Women, L264 slide series through 1998, Slide 3. Source: http://www.cdc.gov/nchstp/hiv_aids/graphics/images/l264/l264-3.htm
4. CDC Pediatric HIV/AIDS Surveillance, L262 slide series through 1998, Slide 9. Source: http://www.cdc.gov/nchstp/hiv_aids/graphics/images/l262/l262-9.htm
5. Centers for Disease Control and Prevention, *HIV/AIDS Surveillance Report, 1999*; 11 (No.1): Table 5. Source: http://www.cdc.gov/nchstp/hiv_aids/stats/hasrlink.htm
6. Centers for Disease Control and Prevention, *HIV/AIDS Surveillance Report, 1999*; 11 (No.1): Table 9. Source: http://www.cdc.gov/nchstp/hiv_aids/stats/hasrlink.htm
7. CDC HIV/AIDS Surveillance—General Epidemiology, L178 slide series through 1998, Slide 7. Source: http://www.cdc.gov/nchstp/hiv_aids/graphics/images/l178/l178-7.htm

8. Healthy People 2010, Draft for Public Comment, September 15, 1998. Source: http://www.health.gov/hpcomments/2010Draft/scripts/fullsearch.cfm
9. Ibid.
10. Ibid.
11. Ibid.
12. Ibid.
13. Ibid.
14. CDC website, Health Topics A–Z: "Chlamydia Facts." Source: www.cdc.gov/nchstp/dstd/chlamydia_facts.htm

TEN

Substance Abuse

NATHAN ERRS IN JUDGMENT

Nathan worked at a local newspaper as a reporter. After work each day, before heading home to his wife and children, he always stopped at the local bar where he would meet some of his friends. It was a bright part of his day. At the time, Nathan thought of himself as a social drinker: "Just a few drinks with the gang and then I'd head home for a late dinner," he recalled. "I never thought the alcohol really affected me."

That innocence ended one evening when, after his normal three double scotches, Nathan headed home as a light rain began to fall. Just a few blocks from his house, heading south, he ran a red light. An eastbound car sideswiped him. Nathan's car spun around, hit a parked car, and then landed on the porch of a neighbors' home. When the police arrived, they administered a sobriety test. Nathan failed.

Fortunately, no one was hurt. But the incident was a wake-up call for Nathan. For a while he worried and fretted, and tried to lie to himself. After all, anyone could make a mistake like that…it was raining…visibility was poor. But in the end he saw no way around the harsh truth: he admitted he was an alcoholic and joined Alcoholics Anonymous. Nathan now has been a member for years and he hasn't had a drop in all that time, but he knows that there is no such thing as an ex-alcoholic. He will always be recovering, but never cured.

WHAT IS SUBSTANCE ABUSE?

In 1990 the Institute of Medicine estimated that approximately one American in every thirty-five over the age of twelve has at some time used illicit drugs. Further, almost all Americans are guilty of substance abuse of some kind or another. Think of all people you know who have to have a cup of coffee in the morning to get themselves going or a pill at night to get to sleep. We are constantly inundated with advertisements for beer, caffeine, pain-killers, cigarettes. We're constantly being told that we just need that "little something"— whether it's a cigarette, drug or drink—and all our problems will be solved. What these ads fail to tell you is that there's no quick fix. Unless you feel good about yourself, and respect yourself enough to treat your body right, your problems will persist.

Simply put, substance abuse is the misuse or non-medical use of drugs, alcohol, or tobacco products. We are guilty of abuse whenever we use substances to alter our moods, self-perceptions, or environments. The specific notion of addiction is a more or less modern one, formulated by Dr. Benjamin Rush in 1790, at a time when the narcotic opium was widely used. The concept is a simple one: Abuse becomes addiction when you develop a physical or psychological dependency on your substance of choice. If you find yourself thinking, "I just have to have one more cigarette, cup of coffee...drink...joint...or upper," then there's a good chance you're an addict.

No matter what you're addicted to, breaking yourself of a habit is never easy. At the same time, it is possible—witness the millions who have kicked theirs. Breaking a habit requires that you be patient with yourself, set small, attainable goals, and take it day by day, hour by hour, minute by minute. Further, when you're trying to break yourself of an addiction, professional help is often necessary. There are many resources available to make your challenge easier. Remember—you are not alone.

Anyone can be a substance abuser. Everyone is at risk, whether black, white, male, female, old, middle-aged or a child in elementary school. Professionals, blue-collar workers, athletes, movie stars, the poor and the rich—all these people fit the profile. In fact, contrary to common belief, approximately 70 percent of all substance abusers are employed. What all this boils down to is that the effects of substance abuse are tearing apart our workplaces, homes, schools, and families.

Substance abuse begins for many different reasons. Some of us turn to alcohol or drugs at a young age because of peer pressure. We all know how difficult it can be to say no when we're trying to feel accepted by the very people who are pushing us to do something. Later, as adults, we may turn to a substance to ease ourselves of depression, mental anguish, or pressure from home or work. 1 Some of us may turn to drugs like amphetamines (speed) to keep us "up," believing that the drug will make us more productive at work. Still others of us, like Nathan, may turn to alcohol or some other drug because it helps us relax and socialize.

Choosing whether to take drugs or use tobacco is a decision we each must make at some time or another. We may rationalize that the substances we use affect only us; therefore, it's no one else's business. However, everyone is at risk when, like Nathan, you get behind the wheel of a car after drinking, or when a drug addict turns to crime to support his or her habit, or when a smoker puts his family at risk of lung cancer because of second-hand smoke. As much as we may want to think so, our bad habits are rarely just our own business.

SUBSTANCE ABUSE AND BLACKS

As within every community, abuse of alcohol and drugs creates great problems within the black community. You know what they are. We've all seen the terrible harvest of physical and mental health problems, lack of education, unemployment, crime, and violence that can be traced back to one cause: a life derailed by substance abuse.

The medical consequences of substance abuse among black people can be terrible: two blacks to every one white die from cirrhosis of the liver, which is caused primarily by alcoholism.[1] Blacks between the ages of 25 and 34 have a 10 percent greater chance of dying from cirrhosis than their white counterparts.[2] Black men die three times more often than white men from esophageal cancer, which is sometimes believed to be caused by the combined abuse of alcohol and tobacco.

"Blacks are three times more likely to be in treatment for a drug abuse-related problem than whites," reads the Report of the Secretary's Task Force on Black and Minority Health, using data obtained from a National Drug and Alcoholism Treatment

Utilization Survey (NDATUS).[3] The statistics speak for themselves. Alcohol, drug abuse, and tobacco use are practically tearing the black community apart.

Nationwide, however, substance abuse seems to be declining somewhat. This may be because the social climate has changed greatly from the late sixties and seventies. Statistics released from the Third Triennial Report to Congress from the Secretary, Department of Health and Human Services on Drug Abuse and Drug Abuse Research indicate that drug use in the United States, while still high, has decreased sharply from the epidemic levels seen in the 1970s. For example:

- Marijuana has been used, at some time or another, by a third of all Americans.[4]

  In 1994, 38% of all high school students had tried marijuana by their senior year, though the same percentage perceived marijuana use as "risky," according to an NIDA survey. The most popular illicit psychoactive substance, marijuana ranks just below caffeine, nicotine, and alcohol as America's drug of choice.

- In 1997, 12-17 year olds were drinking and smoking less than those of the same age in 1988. Still, however, according to the Center for Disease Control (1996), roughly 3300 children and teenagers (all races combined) become regular smokers per day! The upshot is that 4,500,000 teenagers are curent smokers. Data from the National Household Survey during 1988-96, among the same age group, showed that the incidence of the first time and daily cigarette usage increased by 30 percent and 50 percent respectively.[5]

Approximately 20 percent of that same group of children, aged 12-17, had consumed alcohol in the month preceding the 1997 survey. This is down from 25 percent in 1988, but still not a figure we can be happy about.

• In 1997, the National Household Survey showed that the number of blacks that reported using an illicit drug in the preceding month was 7.1 percent compared to the 5.7 percent of whites reporting usage. Further, blacks are more than 1.5 times more likely to experience a drug-induced death than whites.[6]

ALCOHOL AND BLACKS

When it comes to alcohol problems, blacks are disproportionately affected. Sadly enough, the number of us who have medical problems as a result of heavy drinking has increased in recent years. Years ago, rates of acute and chronic alcohol-related diseases among blacks were lower than or similar to those for whites. Recently, however, these rates have increased. Currently, we are at high risk for developing acute and chronic alcohol-related diseases including alcoholic fatty liver, hepatitis, liver cirrhosis, and esophageal cancer (as mentioned above).[75]

Another major difference in black versus white drinking patterns appears to be the ages at which we begin and stop drinking heavily. Among white males, heavy and problematic drinking is most evident among young men. Black men, on the other hand, are more likely to demonstrate problematic drinking habits in middle age, usually after age 30.

WHAT IS ALCOHOLISM?

A simple definition of alcoholism is addiction to ethyl alcohol. Approximately 10 percent of all drinkers become alcoholics. If you're trying to determine if you are addicted to alcohol, you may find the following medically-defined distinctions helpful.

Occasional drinker: If you are an occasional drinker, you drink alcohol sparingly. Alcohol is not a major part of your life, and as a result, has never been a problem.

Frequent drinker: If you are a frequent drinker, you may have a couple drinks at parties or among friends because it makes you feel good. You rarely, however, drink enough to get drunk. People in this group are sometimes referred to as "social drinkers".

Regular drinker: As a regular drinker, you consider drinking an important part of your life. However, you could give up drinking if necessary.

Heavy drinker: If you're a heavy drinker, alcohol is a problem in your life. This means you are alcohol dependent and cannot easily handle social situations without having a drink. You could give up alcohol only with great difficulty, which means you are prone to becoming an alcoholic. If you fall in this group, it would be worth your while to seek help or try to cut down on your alcohol intake.

Alcoholic: An alcoholic is a heavy drinker who has lost control over his or her alcohol consumption. If you're an alcoholic, you cannot function at work, home, or in a social setting without a drink. You also can't stop at one drink. Your alcohol abuse may change your personality drastically, and even cause you to have blackouts on occasion. You may even have lost interest in eating or suffer from severe weight loss. It's important to realize that the effects of alcoholism differ among alcoholics, depending on body chemistry or eating habits.

If you are an alcoholic, a constant threat in your life may be alcohol withdrawal. In other words, if you go too long without having a drink, or if you're trying to become sober or break the addiction, you may experience the "shakes," or hallucinations. During the hallucinations, called delirium tremens, or DTs, you may imagine that you see insects, spiders or other bugs creeping on you. You may also imagine that there are animals in the room with you, probably because you misinterpret shadows and sounds. People may tell you that you're talking compulsively or indistinctly, and your arms and legs may shake, because of muscle twitches and spasms.

These symptoms may be caused by an altered brain function brought about by alcohol abuse, especially among those who have been excessive and steady drinkers for many years, or who are recovering from a recent drinking binge. Current research suggests that DTs may result from a biochemical disorder in the brain.

Sometimes DT symptoms may be accompanied by fever that can get high enough to cause the circulatory system to collapse. About 15 percent of those who experience DTs die because of shock or circulatory collapse. DTs are considered to be a medical emergency. If you experience DTs or are ever with someone who does, seek medical assistance immediately. Large amounts of water are often given intravenously so that the sodium, potassium and magnesium added to it can replace those minerals lost in the perspiration that accompanies high fever. Muscle tremors may be treated with tranquilizing drugs. DTs usually end within approximately two days.

Alcoholism not only affects us physically but also has severe social consequences. Recent statistics show that driving under the influence of alcohol accounts for half of all fatal motor vehicle accidents in the United States. An increasing number of reported industrial accidents, crimes of violence against adults and children, house break-ins, and robberies involve alcohol use. In addition, the number of juvenile alcoholics seems to be increasing. These youngsters, as well as adults, also mix alcohol with other drugs-especially cocaine.

TREATING THE ALCOHOLIC

According to Peter Bell, the director of the Institute on Black Chemical Abuse in Minneapolis, black individuals and families tend to seek help for alcoholic problems later in the progression of the illness than their white counterparts. As a consequence, black families may be significantly more dysfunctional and resistant to messages of recovery than white families.

One comprehensive recovery program designed specifically for the African American Alcoholic can be found in Williams' and Gorski's 1997 publication, *Relapse Prevention Counseling for African Americans, 1997* (Independence Press). This brief (110 pp.) book outlines a step by step approach to recovery.

Alcoholics Anonymous (AA) is one group that tries to help alcoholics help themselves. The philosophy of this group is that "once an alcoholic, always an alcoholic," but that you can control the disease through determination, the support of other recovering alcoholics and, of course, by not drinking. AA has developed Twelve Steps (see below) and a buddy system to help you to sobriety. There are also several groups that have been developed for relatives or friends of alcoholics. These include Al-Anon and Alateen, a program for teenagers whose parents are alcoholics.

Twelve Steps

The following Twelve Steps are established by Alcoholics Anonymous. Millions of Americans have found that by making these steps a way of life, they have been able to break their addiction. No matter what you are addicted to, you may find them to be helpful.

1. We admitted we were powerless over alcohol -that our lives had become unmanageable.

2. Came to believe that a Power greater than ourselves could restore us to sanity.

3. Made a decision to turn our will and our lives over to the care of God as we understood God to be.

4. Made a searching and fearless moral inventory of ourselves.

5. Admitted to God, to ourselves and to another human being the exact nature of our wrongs.

6. Were entirely ready to have God remove all these defects of character.

7. Humbly asked God to remove our shortcomings.

8. Made a list of all persons we had harmed, and became willing to make amends to them all.

9. Made direct amends to such people wherever possible, except when to do so would injure them or others.

10. Continued to take personal inventory and when we were wrong promptly admitted it.

11. Sought, through prayer and meditation, to improve our conscious contact with God as we understood God to be, praying only for knowledge of God's will for us and the power to carry that out.

12. Having had a spiritual awakening as the result of these Steps, we tried to carry this message to others, and to practice these principles in all our affairs.[86]

TOBACCO ABUSE

Another common substance that is abused in American society, especially among blacks, is tobacco. For more information about nicotine addiction, see Chapter Two.

Our fascination with tobacco dates way back. During his explorations, Columbus first discovered Caribbean Indians smoking leaves of the "tabaca" plant and brought the plant back to Europe. In less than 50 years, people in every major city in Europe were smoking. As early as the 1600s, governments attempted to ban the habit, and in some countries the punishment for smoking was death. Yet even with that ultimate discouragement, the number of smokers increased.

Today, 60 million Americans smoke cigarettes and more than 6 million U.S. men smoke cigars. The Report of the Secretary's Task Force on Black Minority Health states that "cigarette smoking is the chief preventable cause of death in the United States. Cigarette smoking is a causal factor for coronary heart disease and arteriosclerotic peripheral vascular disease; cancer of the lung, larynx, oral cavity and esophagus; and chronic bronchitis and emphysema. It is also associated with cancer of the urinary tract, bladder, pancreas, and kidney and with ulcer disease and low birthweight." According to current estimates (Schwabel, 2000), some 430,000 Americans die each year from cigarette smoking, the largest portion of these deaths being cardiovascular.

In April 1993, the Centers for Disease Control and Prevention reported that a steady 25-year decline in smoking had leveled off. The CDC reported that 46.3 million adults (25.7 percent) smoked in 1991, compared to 25.5 percent who smoked in 1990. Their report also stated that more blacks (29.2 percent, versus 26.2 percent in 1990) smoke than any other groups. The age at which someone first takes up smoking is crucial, according to the September 1990 issue of the Journal of the American Medical Association (JAMA). Once you become an established smoker, quitting is more difficult, because nicotine is a highly addictive drug.

According to the JAMA article, which looked at 14,764 people ranging from ages 18 to 35 (of that group, 811 were black men), smoking begins in all racial groups as early as age nine. The incidence of starting to smoke then increases rapidly after age 11, peaking between ages 17 and 19 among all race and ethnic groups. In addition, smoking rates were generally higher for black and Hispanic men and women.[97]

CURTIS LISTENS TO REASON

Curtis is 70 years old and in excellent health. He's up every day at 7 A.M. for a three-mile walk. His neighbors recognize him by his white, blue and purple jumpsuit.

Fifteen years ago, Curtis could barely walk up the six steps to his bedroom in his split-level home.

He smoked two packs of cigarettes a day. During a routine physical, his doctor took X rays of his lungs. The film showed lung damage, the result of 35 years of smoking. Dr. Williams told Curtis that if he didn't stop smoking, he would shorten his life considerably. It was not the first time she had told him this, but it was the first time he listened.

Previously, in Chapter Two, we mentioned the hazardous effects of smoking on the body. About 1 in 5 deaths from cardiovascular diseases are attributable to smoking.

Today, it is estimated that 28.8 percent of all black men and 23.5 of all black women smoke. Though the percentage of black men that smoke has decreased in recent years, black males still smoke at a higher percentage than white males (27.1 per cent).[11]

SMOKELESS TOBACCO

Smokeless tobacco use increased 40 percent between 1970 and 1986 and is used predominately by young men, according to Healthy People 2000. Although statistics show that black men use smokeless tobacco less than whites, it's important to be aware of the risks involved with smokeless tobacco.

Oral cancer appears to occur several times more frequently among smokeless tobacco users than among non- users, and may be 50 times as frequent among long-term snuff users. These very high risks may be the result of the multitude of toxins found in smokeless tobacco. In addition, all smokeless tobacco products contain substantial amounts of nicotine, which may lead to nicotine dependence and eventual cigarette use.[12]

TREATMENT

If you don't smoke, don't start. If you smoke, stop! There are several methods of stopping smoking, such as nicotine patches, self-help classes and hypnosis, among others. Ask your doctor for specific information on how you can stop smoking. Your success relies entirely on your willingness to quit. Attitude is everything. (Refer to Chapter Two for more information about how to break your nicotine addiction.)

OTHER KINDS OF SUBSTANCE ABUSE

While alcohol and nicotine abuse may be most obvious in today's society because they are legal substances, there are many other substances whose abuse have far-reaching consequences for the black community.

EUGENE'S STORY

Eugene is a 28-year-old man who worked 12 to 16 hours a day. He had just finished law school and had been hired by a high-powered law firm that required him to produce approximately 200 billable hours a month. Eugene expected to have to work a lot at first, so he didn't complain.

At the end of his first year at the firm, Eugene and his wife, Delia, purchased a four-bedroom home in an upscale suburban community outside Chicago. He also bought Delia a new Saab. "I earned a great deal of money working all those hours," said Eugene, "but Delia and I were also spending money at a rapid rate. That made me want to work more hours, spending more nights and weekends at work."

The long hours soon began to take a toll on Eugene. He was tired all of the time and even found himself nodding off at social functions. *"I was working on a Fortune 500 account when I started taking uppers to stay awake. One of the associates at my office gave me some during a particularly hairy week. I had been given a chance to prove myself by defending one of our big clients in court. I spent nearly the whole week at work, working all night and dozing off at embarrassing times during the day. I took the pills—I didn't want to lose the account or the case."* Eugene didn't lose either one, but nearly lost Delia after he continued to take amphetamines every day. *"It had gotten to a point where I couldn't function without the pills,"* Eugene said.

DRUGS

When the term drug abuse is mentioned, the assumption is usually that the drug being abused is illegal. Not true. The abuse of prescription drugs is as frequent as the abuse of illegal drugs.

Drug abuse is the misuse or non-medical use of drugs for the purpose of altering your mood or perception. While certain drugs are prescribed by doctors to make you feel better, many illegal drugs attack your central nervous system and cause mental instability and emotional dependency. With some drugs, physical dependency even occurs. These drugs alter your normal behavior.

Following are some of the more common types of illegal drugs that are abused.

Marijuana

Indian hemp has been known to us for at least 3,000 years. Hemp was first used for commercial purposes, such as the production of rope and textiles. It is mentioned in ancient Sanskrit literature dating from 2000 to 1400 B.C. Later, it was utilized for medicinal and anesthetic purposes by Chinese, Hindu and Arab physicians. Not until the tenth century of the Christian era was hemp used extensively, in India and Arab countries, for its intoxicant and euphoric properties.

Among the numerous forms of the drug are Indian hemp, hashish and marijuana. You may have heard marijuana cigarettes referred to as "reefers," "joints," "weed," "grass," or "sticks."

One reason why marijuana in all its forms can have such a potent effect on the user is that it acts not only on the lower brain but also on the cerebral cortex and hippocampus, both of which directly regulate our emotions.

Whether marijuana is physiologically addictive, in the way that heroin or alcohol or nicotine are addictive, is a question still under debate. But most agree that it can be psychologically addictive. Indeed, there are many known cases in which marijuana has triggered psychotic symtoms such as auditory and visual hallucinations, paranoia and'or delusions.

Whatever it's called, marijuana is a depressant that affects your central nervous system. After using marijuana, you might feel sedated, depressed, or drowsy. At the same time, marijuana is sometimes classed as a hallucinogen, because it can affect the mind. Like LSD, though not as strongly, marijuana can cause distorted perceptions, depersonalization, increased sensitivity to sound, and heightened suggestibility. Marijuana can be taken by mouth, baked in a cake or brownies, or smoked, which is the preferred method in the United States. Marijuana cigarettes are most often hand-rolled in white or brown cigarette papers. A heavy user may smoke as many as six cigarettes a day.

When first using marijuana, you likely noticed an increase in your hunger or desire for sweets. As a regular user, you may experience the "munchies" throughout the day. Other side effects include clumsiness and poor coordination, flushing of your face and dilation of your pupils. After smoking a joint, your pulse rate and blood pressure will elevate and you may need to urinate more often.

It's very difficult to recognize a marijuana user by sight, but the drug's smoke has an easily identifiable, distinctive odor. If you smell this odor, or if someone you know seems "spacey," disconnected, or breaks into fits of inappropriate laughter, it's possible he or she is a marijuana user.

If you are a habitual marijuana user, you probably have little desire to be cured. You may believe that smoking marijuana is neither harmful nor habit-forming. But being addicted to marijuana, like any drug, is very dangerous. It may pose long-term risks to your body and it can negatively impact your relationships with those you care about. You may also find yourself to be more irritable, garrulous and complaining than you were before you began using the drug. In some cases, using marijuana may lead you to use stronger, more addictive drugs.

Phencyclidine: PCP

"Angel dust," "green tea," "peace pill," hog," "busy bee," "cyclone," "mist," "goon," "rocket fuel," "crystal," "super joint," "zombie dust," and "elephant tranquilizer" are just some of the street names for phencyclidine (PCP).

PCP was developed by pharmacologists for use as an anesthetic in surgery. Permission for testing the drug on human subjects was granted in 1963 by the Food and Drug Administration (FDA). Though PCP functioned well in the operating room, the aftermath of the drug was terrible. When patients regained consciousness they were disoriented, delirious, hallucinating and depressed. Because of these very serious effects, the FDA withdrew its approval for use with humans. It was approved, however, as an animal anaesthetic.

The prevalence of PCP use is unclear because a wide array of drugs are laced with it. What is clear, however, is that PCP is a neurologically potent drug that blocks neuronal transmission. Again, its effects can be devestating. There are people who never recovered normalcy after using it.

PCP has been on the streets since 1967, when laboratories were set up to produce the drug illegally. PCP is cheap to make, and profits are high. The drug can be taken in three forms: pill, powder or liquid. One drug-abuse expert has called PCP "a drug of terror." In small doses, it gives you a free-floating feeling or numbness, the illusion that your mind has separated from your body. In large doses, it produces symptoms of schizophrenia, which can lead to suicide and violence. The drug is stored in the fat tissues of your brain, and the rate of its breakdown in your liver is very slow.

In addition to hallucinations and flashbacks, PCP can cause drowsiness, an inability to verbalize thoughts, and difficulty in thinking. Profuse sweating, involuntary eye movement, loss of feeling of pain, double vision, lack of muscular coordination, dizziness, nausea and vomiting are all common signs of PCP use.

Lysergic acid diethylamide: LSD

LSD made its appearance in 1943. It was popularized in the sixties, almost single handedly, by Timothy Leary, a young Harvard instructor at the time. Leary preached that LSD "expanded one's consciousness." In 1966, as a result of public outcry, Sandoz Laboratories stopped manufacturing the drug, but it continued to be manufactured illegally. Today, there are no firm figures about the prevalence of LSD use, though a poll in 1990 found that 17% of undergraduates at Tulane University had tried it.[13]

LSD is colorless, odorless, and tasteless. A drop of LSD (too small to be seen without a magnifying glass) is all it takes to cause you to hallucinate. Also known by the nicknames acid, paper, cubes, trips, pearly gates, and heavenly blue, orange sunshine, purple haze, and sunshine, LSD is usually dropped onto a sugar cube or a small square of paper, or is added to orange juice. LSD can also be mixed with inert materials and formed into small tablets or caplets.

Shortly after you ingest LSD, you'll begin to experience physical changes. Your pupils may dilate, heart may palpitate, blood pressure may elevate and the smooth muscles of your internal organs may contract.

At first, these symptoms may seem mild. After 30 minutes, however, you will probably begin to have hallucinations. A hallucinogenic "trip" can last up to 10 hours. The horror of LSD is that, if you use it, you are not in control of yourself. You lose your good judgment, and your environment begins to seem unreal. Some users, feeling indestructible, do foolish things while on a "trip." Your mood may fluctuate when under the influence of LSD, so that you feel happy at ONE moment and then, a minute later, fall into a deep depression.

Barbiturates

In recent years, more and more drug users have become addicted to barbiturates because of their relatively easy availability, as compared to opiates and marijuana. Opiate addicts frequently use barbiturates to tide them over when opiates are either unobtainable or in short supply. Like chronic alcoholics, barbiturate addicts may use the drug for a single night's binge, for prolonged sprees, or every day for months or years. In many cases, people use barbiturates along with alcohol or amphetamines. Barbiturate addicts seem to prefer the more potent, rapidly active drugs, such as Nembutal and Seconal. General terms for barbiturates are "goof balls" and "barbs." You may have also heard them referred to as "yellow jackets" or "pink ladies"—special terms that correspond to the color of the capsules.

Barbiturate users generally take 1.0 to 1.5 grams daily, usually orally, though some addicts prefer the intravenous route. Barbiturates can be extremely irritating and may cause large pus pockets if injected into subcutaneous tissues (just under the skin).

TYRONE SELLS DRUGS

Tyrone began selling drugs when he was in his teens to support himself, his mother, and his two sisters. He was a very likable young man and his teachers did everything to convince him to stay in school, but he dropped out when his father deserted his family. He found a job in the neighborhood grocery store as a butcher, but "It didn't pay enough," he said. "I made more money selling drugs for a few hours than cutting meat for a week.

"My mother didn't like it but there was nothing she could do about it," Tyrone said. His mother worked as a cleaning woman in a downtown office building. Tyrone told his mother that he would

stop selling drugs as soon as the family was out of debt and they could get a nice place to live.

Tyrone was now a "businessman." He wore tailored suits and Italian shoes.

His hands were manicured, and he drove a midnight blue convertible. He moved his mother into a new home, and he married a beautiful young woman. Soon, Tyrone was managing a fairly large shopping center, and he and his wife were expecting their first child. He had not given up his drug connections. In fact, the scenario got worse because, in addition to selling, Tyrone had started using cocaine. It was difficult to be around it and not try it, Tyrone says now. So he tried it and got hooked.

"It took the birth of my daughter to make me realize what I was doing to my body and my family," Tyrone said. "My wife wouldn't let me near the baby. My nose was running, my speech was slurred, my eyes were red and I couldn't perform in the bedroom."

Tyrone became determined to get away from his drug connections and make a new life for himself and his family. He moved his family to another state where he spent three months in a treatment program. He is now a manager of a family-owned business and counsels young adults against the use of drugs.

Heroin

Heroin is a narcotic that comes from opium. An opiate (morphine or codeine, for example) is a drug that causes sleep or stupor, and at the same time relieves pain. Be- cause opiate drugs make people insensitive to pain, they are known by the medical community as analgesic drugs and by others as pain killers. Some of the street names for heroin are "H," "skag," "junk," "dirt," "boy," "horse," "smack," "Mexican mud," and "brown sugar."

The only natural source of morphine and codeine is opium. Opium comes from the poppy plant, which thrives in the hot, dry climates of Turkey, China, India, Iran and Mexico. Heroin is a semi-synthetic drug made from the morphine obtained from the stem of the poppy. At one time, heroin addicts were thought to be found only in poor economic areas in large inner cities. But heroin has moved from ghetto alleys to upper-middle- class living rooms and the kitchens of small-town America. An investor can buy a huge amount of heroin for $1,000 in France, and then sell it wholesale in the U.S. for more than $1 million.

Heroin is usually injected into your veins, which is called "mainlining." "Skin-popping" is when you inject the liquid form of the drug under your skin. Heroin may also be taken into your body through your nose, which is known as "snorting." The user's goal is to allow the heroin to travel through his or her bloodstream, so that it reaches all cells in the body. Heroin use affects your brain cells and decreases your heartbeat and respiration rate. Have you ever wondered why heroin addicts often wear dark sunglasses, even at night? The pupils of their eyes dilate and constrict because of the rise and fall of heroin in the blood. They wear glasses to hide this inappropriate dilation of their pupils.

Heroin is a highly addictive narcotic. If you are addicted to heroin, you are probably mentally and physically incapable of thinking or doing anything without the drug. It takes larger and larger doses to get the same effect, and you can become painfully ill with muscle cramps and vomiting when you do not have access to the drug.

You can tell if someone is addicted to heroin if they frequently nod off or are drowsy. This will be especially evident right after they've had a "fix." Another dead giveaway is needle tracks along arms, hands and legs. Addicts may also frequently experience ulcerated sores from using dirty needles or from contaminants in the heroin.

Malnutrition is a serious consequence of heroin addiction. If you are addicted, food will not appeal to you. Your only interest will be the drug. You will probably lose a great deal of weight and become very susceptible to disease. Because heroin addicts use and share dirty needles, it is also not uncommon for them to suffer from blood poisoning, hepatitis, malaria and AIDS. (See Chapter Nine for more information on AIDS.)

Cocaine

The Incas of Peru were the first civilization to record their use of cocaine. They called it "the gift from God." At that time, cocaine use meant the chewing of the leaf. The Incas would do this from day break until sun-down.

Whatever cocaine may have been for the Incas, the form of cocaine used by our civilization has been no gift. We might more aptly call it a curse—a curse that has worsened over the years. In the 60s and early 70s, cocaine use was confined to the white middle class. When crack came along in the eighties, the drug became cheaper, more widely available, and more dangerous. Between 1984-87, for instance, 18% of New York City motor vehicle fatalities were found, upon autopsy, to have ingested significant levels of cocaine.[14]

Cocaine-related deaths among blacks have increased over the past years. Cocaine addiction is very hard to break. Just as with heroin, cocaine will cause you to "lose your conscience." If you are addicted to cocaine, you are likely to do anything to get more of the drug. Mothers who are addicted often forget to take care of their children. Addicts will give up their homes, jobs and families—getting more of the drug is their only concern.

Street names for cocaine are "coke," "snow," "snowbirds," "C", "happy dust," "gold dust," "flake," "Cecil," "stardust", "Bernice," "white girl," "girl," and "speedball" (which is heroin and cocaine together). Cocaine is an odorless, sometimes crystalline or fluffy white powder. Unlike heroin or morphine it is a stimulant. This means instead of making you sleepy, it will keep you awake. Cocaine is usually taken into your bloodstream by one of four methods, snorting, mainlining, smoking, or "skin pops." When you "snort", or take cocaine through your nose, its effect lasts a long time. When you inject it into your bloodstream through mainlining the effect of the drug lasts for approximately 10 minutes. It is possible for IV drug abusers to "use up" all the veins in their body through overuse. When this happens, some abusers will become so desperate that they'll do "skin pops," which means they inject the drug under the skin into capillaries just beneath the skin's surface.

Cocaine base can also be smoked, which is called "freebasing." To process cocaine hydrochloride for freebasing, the drug is treated with a solution of baking soda and ether. When these are mixed together, a layer of liquid containing cocaine forms on the top. This layer is removed into a separate dish, and the extra liquid is allowed to evaporate. The powder produced by this process is known as "freebase." It is put into a water pipe and heated with a propane torch to turn the cocaine into vapor. It was once publicized that comedian Richard Pryor was badly burned from an explosion of ether as he was preparing to freebase.

To avoid the inconvenience and danger of preparing cocaine for freebasing, chemists who deal in illegal drugs have developed a simpler method of changing cocaine hydrochloride into a smokable form. The result is a new drug called "crack." (See next section.)

Regardless of how you take it, cocaine works on your central nervous system, raising your pulse and respiration rates, increasing your body temperature, and elevating your blood pressure. Cocaine constricts your blood vessels and dilates your pupils. The drug induces a kind of hyperactive state, which can bring about a euphoria that seems initially to stimulate your sexual desire. With long-term, chronic use, however, the drug can cause you to lose interest in sex altogether or to become impotent.

Continued use of cocaine is damaging, and the symptoms of chronic cocaine abuse are serious. If you use cocaine, you can experience delusions of persecution, grandeur, jealousy, or violence. You may also experience muscle spasms. If you use cocaine often, you will probably be constantly nervous, excitable, oversensitive to noise and susceptible to frequent mood swings, memory loss, compulsive scribbling (graphomania), and anxiety. You may suffer from auditory and visual hallucinations that make you think someone is persecuting or oppressing you. If you are a chronic user, you can be very dangerous to those around you, and may be capable of committing brutal crimes, or may even attempt suicide or homicide. In addition to mental disturbances, you may develop such physiological disorders as feebleness, emaciation, digestive disorders, nausea, vomiting, loss of appetite, a fast pulse, or impotence.

Crack

Crack, as mentioned above, is created from pure cocaine during the freebasing process. Today, it is the drug of choice on the streets of America. Crack is processed in illegal laboratories in "crack houses" by mixing ordinary cocaine with a solution of baking soda or ammonia and then heating it until the water evaporates. The residue from this "cooking" is crack, a solid crystalline substance that is then broken into pieces or chips. Two or three of these chips make a dose of crack, which is sold on the street for $5 to $25.

Crack is taken into your body by smoking the substance from a glass pipe. Many users also crush crack and smoke it like a marijuana joint. When heated, the chips crackle, thus the name "crack." Heating crack changes it to smoke, which is inhaled, drawn into your lungs and then diffused rapidly throughout your blood-stream. Your circulating blood transports the dissolved cocaine to your brain, where it takes effect immediately. Snorted cocaine reaches your brain in two or three minutes, but smoked cocaine reaches your brain in a matter of seconds.

The effect you feel when smoking crack is called a "rush," which is a sudden high caused by the assault on your brain and central nervous system. Under that assault the nervous system responds by stimulating certain body reactions: increased body temperature, involuntary movement of muscles, and over-stimulation of the pleasure centers in your brain. Since the high from crack lasts for a short period, ranging from one to ten minutes, the drug is used up very quickly.

The reason why crack is so addictive is precisely that its effects come so quickly. In the case of oral ingestion (that is, chewing the coca leaf), the effects begin in 5 to 10 minutes. If one snorts cocaine, the high starts in 2-3 minutes. But crack provides the ultimate instant gratification: its initial effects begin with 8-10 seconds.

When the high level of chemical activity in the brain cells stops, a crack user will often experience a condition called a "rebound." A rebound can happen with any form of cocaine. If you feel extremely depressed, lethargic or negative after crack use, there's a good chance you're experiencing a rebound. Too often, that's when users look for another hit.

Even after a short period of time, regular crack use will have abnormal effects on your brain. Your brain's pleasure centers will slow down. As your pleasure centers lose their ability to respond, you may decide to increase your dose of the drug in order to regain your rush or high. The attempt to get pleasure from the drug becomes so compelling that many addicts devote their entire lives to obtaining and smoking crack.

To make matters worse, a combination of cocaine and heroin, called a "speed ball," has become increasingly popular. This deadly combination has resulted in countless deaths, among them, some well-known celebrities.

EFFECTS OF COCAINE AND CRACK

Here are some of the ways cocaine and crack can affect your body:

Blood vessels: Cocaine and crack can increase your blood pressure to such a degree that you can be at risk of having a stroke. In fact, doctors have reported an increasing number of fatal strokes among crack users.

Skin: Occasionally the skin on your face will get oily and become covered with pimples.

Eyes: As with heroin, cocaine and crack cause the pupils of your eyes to dilate and remain open. Your eyes then become sensitive to light and your vision will become impaired during drug use. To reduce these problems, many crack addicts wear dark glasses constantly.

Heart: Using cocaine or crack will speed up your normal heart rate by 30 to 50 percent. Both drugs can also interfere with the regularity of your heartbeat, making it skip a beat and then do two rapid contractions to compensate. It can also cause a heart attack.

Lungs: Cocaine and crack both inhibit the proper exchange of oxygen and carbon dioxide in your body and destroy your lung tissue and air sacs. Users of these drugs often develop bronchitis.

Muscles: Both drugs affect your muscles and cause facial tics or involuntary jerks. You may even suffer from convulsions after using these drugs.

TREATING DRUG ABUSE

If you're a drug user, whether the drug is alcohol, crack or even nicotine, your substance of choice may very well be the most important thing in your life. It's very likely that you don't want to quit. You probably get a lot of pleasure from the way the substance makes your body feel, at least for a while. After all, using drugs and alcohol can be very social. Your friends or family may not think you're being cool if you tell them you want to stop. However, your drug or alcohol use may also be ripping you apart from those who care about you most, those who want you to be healthy and in control.

Regardless of what his situation is, breaking an addiction of any sort could very well be the most difficult thing a man needs to do as a human being. At the same time, when it comes to your health and true happiness, seeking help is the strongest, most courageous thing you can ever do for yourself.

John Lucas is one hero who overcame drug addiction. A former player for the Houston Rockets and a recovering drug addict,

Lucas was given a second chance by the sports world when he was named coach of the San Antonio Spurs basketball team. In this new capacity, Lucas formed a counseling group to help other basketball players and athletes like himself who had been banned from participating in organized sports because of drug use. Today, Lucas uses many of the recovery strategies he learned when fighting his addiction to guide his basketball team to victory.

If you're looking to break your addiction to drugs, you'll be happy to know that you have many different options. Health experts and community service programs, such as Narcotics Anonymous (NA) and Cocaine Anonymous (CA) have developed three approaches to drug treatment: detoxification, maintenance and therapeutic communities.

- *Detoxification* means that you're taken off the drug as soon as possible. Your physical and psychological distress resulting from the withdrawal process is then treated.

- *Maintenance* usually means you are given a synthetic narcotic (methadone), which mimics the effects of the drug you have been using, but does not have the same side effects. The replacement synthetic drug allows you to wean yourself off the drug without the trauma of going "cold turkey," or stopping drug use immediately. This treatment is only effective if you are addicted to a narcotic.

- Entering a *therapeutic community* is one way drug addicts have been able to successfully recover. In 1958, a former alcohol and drug addict, Chuck Dedrich, set up a new type of treatment center for drug addicts. He called it Synanon and modeled it, on Alcoholics Anonymous, of which he had been a member. There are now more than 300 such centers throughout the country. Addicts at Synanon are called clients because they or someone else pays for the treatment, and all members enter the program voluntarily. Most clients are from a minority group; quite often they come from unstable homes, many are poorly educated. The staff of Synanon is composed of ex-addicts, counselors and other trained professionals.

CONCLUSION

The effects of substance abuse can be devastating—both to you, if you're an abuser, and to your friends, family and coworkers. If your life is so stressful or unpleasant that you must rely on a substance to cope, try to deal with the cause of the tension in another way. Sports, exercise, or stress-reduction techniques can all help. Sometimes opening up to a family member, a close friend or even a therapist can help you find the support you need to make a change.

Abuse of any kind is hard to break, and finding the support you need is essential. If you are a substance abuser, remember you are not alone. Not only are there thousands of people in the same situation as you, there is also a network of confidential professionals who are willing to help. Take it day by day and set small goals for yourself. Seek assistance and reach out to your family and friends who care and are willing to offer guidance and support. You may be surprised how helpful others will be.

Your ultimate success will be up to you. You owe it to yourself to lead a long, healthy and happy life. Make a choice to give yourself the greatest gift you can ever give: health. Step by step, you can break your addiction. You just have to make the first move.

RESOURCES

Al-Anon
One Park Avenue
New York, NY 10016 (800) 356-9996
*(Al-Anon provides information and support for families of alco-
holics, using the 12-Step program.)*

Alcoholics Anonymous
P.O. Box 459
Grand Central Station
New York, NY 10017 (212) 870-3400
*(AA offers brochures, pamphlets and self help for those interested
in recovery. You can find your local chapter in the white pages of
your telephone book.)*

American Cancer Society
777 Third Avenue
New York, NY 10017
(212) 586-8700
(800) 422-6237
(The Society offers free information, literature, and referrals.)

American Health Foundation
320 East 42nd Street
New York, NY 10595
(212) 953-1900
(The Foundation offers self-help brochures.)

American Lung Association
1740 Broadway
New York, NY 10019-4374 (212) 315-8700
(The Association offers materials on smoking classes, as well as general pamphlets and brochures. Look up your local association office in your telephone book.)

The Hazelden Foundation
Hazelden Education Materials
Center City, MN., 55012.
(The Hazeldon Foundation publishes a number of excellent pamphlets on substance abuse treatment and recovery. You can write to them for titles.)

National Clearinghouse for Alcohol and Drug Abuse Information
Box 2345
Rockville, MD 20850
(301) 468-2600
(800) 729-6686
(The Clearinghouse offers brochures and pamphlets free to the public. Ask for their most recent catalogue of free publications. You can also speak to a specialist about any specific problems.)

NOTES FOR CHAPTER 10

1. Herd, Denise, "Migration, Cultural Transformation and the Rise of Black Cirrhosis," paper presented at the Alcohol Epidemiology Section, Internation Council on Alcohol and Addictions, Padova, Italy, June 1983.
2. Secretary's Task Force on Black and Minority Health, 8 vols. (Washington, D.C.: United States Department of Health and human Services, 1985), 1:70-75

3. Ibid., p. 136.
4. "The Third Triennial Report to Congress from the Secretary, Department of Health and Human Services on Drug Abuse and Drug Abuse Research," 1991, pp. 2-3.
5. U.S. Department of Health and Human Services, Healthy People 2010 (Conference Edition, in Two Volumes). Washington, D.C.: January 2000
6. U.S. Department of Health and Human Services, Healthy People 2010.
7. Ibid., pp. 33-34.
8. "The Twelve Steps and Traditions," Al-Anon Family Groups (1973), New York, p. 2.
9. Escobedo, Luis G.; Anda, Robert F.; and Mast, Eric E. (1990) "Sociodemographic Characteristics of Cigarette Smoking Initiation in the United States," IJAMA, September 26, 1990, vol. 264, no. 12, 1550-54.
10. American Heart Association, 2000 Heart and Stroke Statistical Update. Dallas, Tex.: American Heart Association, 1999, p. 20.
11. American Heart Association, Biostatistical Fact Sheets [On-line]/ Available FTP: Host name american heart.org Directory: Heart_and_Stroke_A__Z Guide/cigs.
12. "New Reports Make Recommendations, Risk for Resources to Step TB Epidemic," IJAMA,I January 13, 1933, vol. 269, no. 2, pp. 187-188,
13. L. Johnson, et al., Monitoring the Future, Vol II, 1975-66. NIH, 1996
14. P. M. Marzuk, et al., "Prevalence of Recent Cocaine Use Among Motor Vehicle Fatalities in N. Y.," JAMA, 1990; 250-56.

ELEVEN

Violence

JASON AND DARNEL'S STORY

Jason and Darnel have a lot in common. They're both intelligent, energetic, and fun to be around. They have much to give, and their most productive years are ahead of them. Unfortunately, they also share a disability: Both of them are now wheelchair bound because they were each shot in the back.

Jason comes from a large family with four brothers and two sisters. Jason's mother and father both work full time. By saving and carefully managing their money, they were able to buy a home and move out of the projects when Jason was just seven years old. Jason was known as a talker. He was engaging and at times wise beyond his years, and he could captivate older folk with ease. Some people felt he talked too much, but that was just the way he was.

Jason was extremely close to his best friend, Darnel. Their personalities, though, were complete opposites: whereas Jason was outgoing, a talker, Darnel's friends described him as cool and in control. He expressed himself well but was usually brief and to the point.

271

Darnel's mother and father believed in education. Both of them worked full time and preached to Darnel constantly about bettering himself. He loved sports, excelled in math, and was a big hit with the young ladies of the neighborhood. In fact, both young men were much admired by "the sisters."

THE INCIDENT

The whole thing started over a single marijuana joint. Jason, who'd never smoked, tried it at a party and suddenly got high for the first time. He knew he didn't feel right but couldn't help himself. He started talking loudly and making wild gestures with his hands. Some of his friends, though he hardly noticed, were moving away from him.

What Jason didn't know was that the weed was laced with phencyclidine, also known as PCP. PCP can cause a break with the real world—called a psychotic reaction. Darnel had taken a drag as well, but something warned him to stop, and he didn't take a second one.

Darnel saw the fight begin. Somebody said Jason was bad-mouthing a man neither of them knew. Suddenly, the man was waving a gun. Jason was still shouting at him. As Darnel tried to move in and pull him away, shots were fired, and both friends went down in the melee. Though they survived, both Jason and Darnel were left paralyzed from the waist down.

There is a growing legion of young black men paralyzed and wheelchair bound because of mind-numbing violence like the episode we just witnessed. In most cases, and certainly in this one, these tragedies could have been prevented. Jason and Darnel were experimenting with the wrong thing at the wrong time.

Jason lost control, and both lives were changed forever by one fateful event.

Of course, bad things *do* happen to good people. But many times they don't have to. It's important to understand how the interaction of drugs, parties, friends, acquaintances, and arguments can determine whether a person lives or dies. Young and old people alike should know that alcohol, other drugs, arguments, and tempers mix badly. Although PCP-laced weed was the culprit this time around, alcohol can be equally bad. In fact, alcohol is the drug most commonly associated with murder.

Statistics can't capture the suffering and long-term stress created by these violent acts, or even their frequency. It has been said that for every homicide there are 100 nonfatal assaults, so homicide is just the tip of the iceberg. Something just as frightening lurks just below the surface. Ask Darnel and Jason. And though it may seem as if they have already paid the price for making unwise choices, they will continue to pay as long as they live.

The two men have pressed on with their lives. Darnel goes to college, and Jason works full time—but both carry the wounds of this ongoing American epidemic. Largely ignored by the wider society, young black men have borne the brunt of this fierce destruction for the last 35 years. Why? What conditions create among us an environment where murder and mayhem reign supreme?

HISTORY'S CONTRIBUTION

Though history isn't an excuse for present violent behavior, it is impossible to discuss violence as a health issue without taking a historical perspective. Historically, some of the most brutal and violent acts were committed in America by white men with the support of their friends and families. One need only witness the pictures of the lynchings that took place in the 1930s, 1940s, and 1950s to begin to understand the deep-seated hatred and psychology of oppression that ran rampant in this country. In some cases, women and children witnessed these public killings. (We can only surmise the long-term impact this kind of trauma can have on a child.) Unfortunately, although less common, these kinds of brutality go on even today.

The idea that black men are less than human is certainly suggested by such acts. How else could one person burn another person alive? How else could two white men drag a chained black man behind a pickup truck and drag him to his death? The answer appears to be that if one group of people constantly demonizes another, murders of members of the demonized group seem bearable and even acceptable.

Why does the image of the black man as a demon persist? Is it a question of those in power defining reality as they see it? Is it a vestige of slavery that has yet to be purged from the American mind? Does it serve the purpose of elevating those who are not black to a loftier plane? Whatever the answer, the dehumanization of black men obviously reinforces the message that some people are better than others.

Of course, many black males of stature have weathered personal storms and are looked upon with respect and even idolized by the majority community. However, these people always seem to be viewed as special cases—not to be confused with the majority of blacks, who are said to be irresponsible, inarticulate, and even unintelligent. The media images of black men as minstrels, street pimps, drug addicts, pushers, hustlers, and con-men persist even today.

There seems no cure for this continuing national sickness other than a dialogue between the races—a thoughtful discussion of images, symbols, culture, and heritage that can help us sort out where we continue to go wrong as a nation. The Presidential Commission on Race headed by John Hope Franklin (master teacher and historian) was a step in the right direction, but the dialogue must continue. As things stand, the issue of violence and race remains an unresolved menace for all of us, and no prescription for health will be complete unless this issue is addressed and resolved.

RACISM: THE UNRESOLVED MENACE

All of us are bombarded with images and stereotypes that prevent logical discussion, or even thought, about violence. A young black man, accused of killing a policeman in New Jersey, is brutally beaten in front of his family, jailed, and humiliated, only to be released within a few days as the evidence overwhelming clears him of any wrongdoing. The assistant prosecutor resigns in protest after this man's arrest.

Not even the very celebrities that are held up as exceptions are spared such stereotyping. Danny Glover, a famous black actor, is unable to get a taxicab to stop for him in New York City and is forced to call a news conference to publicly address this situation. We've all seen a rash of false arrests, planted evidence, wrongful convictions, and even murders by the police of African American and Latino American men in major cities throughout the United States.

Governor George Ryan of Illinois recently called for a moratorium on the death penalty because so many death row inmates have been cleared by DNA evidence. Men on death row are primarily black or Latino. In many cities, young African American teenagers are harassed by police every day just because of their race. And once a black male is arrested, there's no guarantee that he'll ever see his family again. The brutal torture of Abner Louima while in police custody clearly demonstrates that black men are physically at risk even after arrest.

A hallmark of the American justice system states that the accused is innocent until proven guilty, but this presumption of innocence doesn't always seem to apply to blacks. Many people living in minority neighborhoods are deeply concerned about police violence. The police slaying of Amadou Diallo and, more recently, of Patrick M. Dorismond in New York City clearly depict the tenuous line blacks walk on a daily basis. There are concerned and caring professional police in this country, but for many people in the black community, these police officers are not often visible.

We can not ignore the contribution of such stereotyping made by the glaring misrepresentation of black men on television, movies, radio, and print media. The image of the angry criminal black male as a public menace remains firmly in the minds of the majority, and helps to explain why an elderly white woman would clutch her purse when a black man enters the elevator she's on. These emotions are best addressed by facts, knowledge, wisdom, and understanding—this is a job that requires the best from people of good will on both sides of the racial line.

We reemphasize that these observations do not excuse criminal behavior or the actions of some black men. *However, the majority of African American men, both young and old, are law abiding and responsible.*

THE PROBLEM WITH ALCOHOL

Records from medical examiners' offices in major cities reveal that alcohol intoxication is a factor in approximately half of all murders. One reason why alcohol-related violence is so sadly common in black and Latino neighborhoods is that alcohol is marketed selectively there. Not long ago, Reverend Calvin Butts, the pastor of Abysinnia Baptist Church in Harlem (and now president of SUNY at Old Westbury), initiated a campaign to rid Harlem of shameless alcohol and tobacco billboards that link alcohol intake with sex, power, and glamour. Reverend Butts's campaign was important because it saw these billboards as an assault on community health. In his view, because each community creates its own collective health, the schools, parks, centers, churches, and playgrounds that make up the community fabric must be protected. It's up to each community to assess threats to its health, whether the threats are unwanted incinerators that release toxic waste or 8-foot billboards that encourage our youth to participate in risky and unhealthy behaviors. Men and women of conscience must stand watch.

THE ART OF HEALTHY CONFRONTATION

Most men have faced some type of fight in their lives, whether on the playground or in the boardroom. There's a great deal on the line when one person delivers a challenge to another. Your whole definition of self can be wrapped up in the confrontation. To back down puts you on the defensive and can open you to further assaults.

That is the dilemma. But happily, as in the case of many dilemmas, solutions become available when we shift our point of view. Part of the solution lies in recognizing limits and boundaries of our actions. Knowing that fighting is only one way to settle a dispute can actually provide a sense of security. Do we really want to enter the realm of accelerating violence and brutal dirty play whose outcome can bring the kinds of results it did for Jason and Darnel? No, for most of us there is much to be said for defusing a potential confrontation.

Here are three ways to practice healthy, as opposed to violent, confrontation.

- *Rough-housing with boundaries*
  People's attempts to intimidate usually begin with words. Some ballplayers like to berate their adversaries by talking trash. But surprisingly and happily, for all the physicality of basketball, football, and soccer, serious, injury-producing fights are rare. What players sometimes *do* practice, as a kind of venting, is "air punching"—that is, they throw punches that aren't directed at anyone in particular. This tactic is a sign that these athletes understand the need for limits and that a challenge doesn't have to mean a fight to the death. The rough-housing that many young males engage in is a way of learning the give and take of life, but with boundaries that prevent serious injury.

- *The martial arts*
  The second way a person can learn to confront constructively is to study the martial arts. Long known as an effective way to increase self-discipline, clear thought, and confidence, the daily practice of these fighting skills is healthy emotionally and physically. (The aerobic conditioning is a special physical benefit.)

One of the basic teachings of most martial arts is the emphasis on self-defense. Indeed, the student of these arts must not be the aggressor. The emphasis is on *avoiding* a fight. If a fight should occur, the goal is to disarm and render the aggressor harmless. In the art of Aikido, the aggressor's energy and force is used to neutralize him. Some Karate "Katas" are specifically designed to concentrate a person's life force, creating around him a sphere of protection and peace. Although it may seem contradictory, studying martial arts can produce a strong commitment to nonviolence—and encourage regular exercise.

- *Civil disobedience*
The third model of healthy confrontation we'll discuss is civil disobedience, which was used so effectively during the struggle for civil rights. The Montgomery Bus Boycott, The Greensboro Lunch Counter sit-ins, and the Mississippi Freedom Rides are historical examples of healthy confrontations initiated to help break the back of segregation and exclusion. These examples remind us that there's a deep tradition of nonviolence in the black community, nurtured in the black church and practiced by young and old alike. The courage and determination of the young people who risked their lives doing freedom work (the Student Non-Violent Coordinating Committee is just one example) can give all of us strength in these days of despair. Some of us are drifting in midlife with little energy and even less resolve. We should examine the historical record carefully because our mental health could be improved if we were to work sincerely for justice. There are life lessons here for us all.

DOMESTIC VIOLENCE: A SILENT STORM

This was the third time Stephanie had been brought to the emergency room, and each time her story was much the same: She had tripped coming down the stairs and bruised herself. The emergency room doctor was suspicious even the first time around. Stephanie's black eyes and neck bruising just didn't fit with this type of fall. Stephanie's husband, Frank, who always accompanied her to the ER, did most of the talking and always seemed to be in too much of a hurry. The third time Frank brought Stephanie to the ER, the doctor asked him to step outside the room. But Frank flatly refused to go, so the doctor failed to get the detailed history he hoped for. Two weeks later, Stephanie was dead—yet another victim of domestic homicidal abuse.

We've shown you a snapshot of a tragedy still all too common in America. Despite increased media exposure, thousands of women continue to suffer at the hands of their spouses, lovers, boyfriends, and ex-partners.

Violence against women knows no racial barrier. Although we don't always know why men become abusers, we have a few answers. Sometimes alcohol plays a role, sometimes stress. Sometimes the man's low sense of self-worth sets the stage for domestic violence.

Though the causes may be varied, it's essential for men to understand that domestic violence against women is *never* the woman's fault. There's no excuse for physically assaulting a woman or emotionally intimidating or brutalizing her. Sure, the woman's behavior may have been irritating. All of us can do irritating things from time to time. But these irritations *never* excuse physical abuse.

Because of the traditional power differences between men and women, women who are victims of domestic violence can feel locked in abusive situations that they can't escape because they lack financial and physical support. At the same time, a woman's hesitance to leave an abusive relationship is sometimes based on another sound fact: More than 40 percent of women who leave abusive relationships face retaliative physical assault and possibly death at the hands of their significant others.

It's clear that men who abuse women need counseling and healing. Often they need distance as well. The wisest thing an abusive man can do is leave home, provide economic support for the woman and children, and stay away until he has control over his emotions and has gotten the help he needs to ensure that he is no longer a threat to others.

Abusive men must acknowledge that they need help and that the problem rests with them alone. The road back can be long and hard. With the help of a counselor or psychiatrist, the abusive man will need anger management sessions, impulse control training, and good counseling to help him gain insight into how this problem began. He may also need to learn to strengthen his own capacity for love and his appreciation of the benefits of a loving relationship. All men, even if they are not abusers, should strive for greater insight into what it means to be a man and into a deeper understanding of their responsibilities in a relationship.

Even outside domestic life, abuse can be a problem. Modern life has created new opportunities for women as well as men. This means that, more than ever before, men and women interact in the workplace. So new issues of abuse and harassment are arising there, too. Black men—indeed all men—must learn how to avoid making offensive and insensitive statements. We all need to cultivate attitudes that help set a healthy tone on the job and at home. Often, it boils down simply to the Golden Rule: If we treat women as we wish to be treated, the rewards on both sides will be plentiful.

PUTTING IT ALL TOGETHER

Black men in America face violence every day. From distorted media images to unwelcome glances of fear or menace, from the sense of being under constant surveillance to black-on-black homicide and police brutality, violence surrounds black males. The fact is, no one who fears for his life or well-being can be deemed healthy.

Because black men have the lowest life expectancy of all groups in America today, we *must* begin to address the epidemic of violence with a major goal in mind: *prevention*. Some of our youth have been seduced by the "gangsta" image—the power and glamour of being admired and feared has captured their imaginations. The violence that surrounds rap singers has become part of the hip-hop scene. For many African American men who wish to emulate them it has also become common behavior. Unfortunately, such a life, based on street violence and vengeance, often leads to death and destruction.

It is up to us to demonstrate another more balanced way in life. We can still celebrate the energy of hip-hop, but without the violent baggage. We can begin to help our young people understand the importance of camaraderie, belonging, respect, standards, and authority. Responsible older men must help nurture the emotional health of younger ones. We can do this through the process of change and development that some people refer to as the "rites of passage." Specifically, we can begin to do this by showing in our words and actions:

- That children are sacred and must be protected. Each child must have an opportunity to grow with proper love, guidance, and support.

- That because of the link between black-on-black violence and alcohol, African American men need to cut back on their alcohol intake and thus reduce the likelihood of tragic alcohol-related violence.

- That because even drugs like marijuana, deemed to be "safe," are often laced with more dangerous chemicals, and because young men are particularly susceptible, we need to explode the "cool" aura often associated with getting high. This means abstaining and teaching others to abstain from crack, cocaine, LSD, and other mind-altering drugs.

- That relationship between men and women depends on mutual trust and respect, and that emotional or physical abuse of women is not a sign of manhood but rather the opposite.

THE IMPORTANCE OF SUPPORT

Some men seem to think that talking about feelings is unmanly. The fact is that all of us need a few close friends with whom we can share difficult issues without being judged. Sometimes we need more. If you feel ready to explode, seek professional help immediately. (A counselor or a psychiatrist is a good place to begin.) Sure, you may feel there's a stigma associated with seeing a psychiatrist. Overcome that fear, keeping in mind that the failure to get help can result in the ruin of your own life and sometimes the life of another. In some cases, a psychiatrist will prescribe for you medication that can help you with anger control. In others, through patient conversation, he or she will help you untie the knots of anger that disable you.

The Surgeon General, Dr. David Satcher, has made mental illness a major focus of his educational program. This program speaks not only to violence against others but also to violence against oneself. The suicide risk among black youth is rising, and we can't stop that rise until we eliminate the stigma attached to emotional disorders. We can all help bring about the changes necessary in order for people who need help most to get it without fear of ridicule.

Some African American fathers need to be more responsible for their kids. Indeed, all responsible African American men must take on themselves the tasks of mentoring young men. This means spending time with them. It means teaching them to cope with stress without turning to violence. And it means showing them the love and acceptance they need more than anything else.

That's a big agenda, and it doesn't end there. Black men must work to rid America of the cancer called racism. This means speaking out against police brutality and harassment, and against society's unequal treatment of blacks even when we try to get loans and obtain credit. The struggle for equal treatment is an essential part of our own health prescription.

Poverty, unemployment, and depressed conditions all help to feed violence, so all Americans must work to eliminate these conditions. The fact is, when blight and despair decrease, violence decreases with them. Simple prescriptions, such as boot camps or curfews, don't address the roots of these problems. The *real* struggle is in the minds of those people most likely to become involved in a violent event.

Finally, one of the most important antiviolence strategies is to control the easy availability of guns in this country.

When all is said and done, we black men must destroy the myths and demand that the truth be told. We must teach our boys how to be men, and we must strive every day to set an example that each of us can be proud of. This is how the epidemic of violence will end.

SUGGESTED READINGS

Frantz Fanon and the Psychology of Oppression, by Hussein Abdilahi Bulhan (Plenum Press, 1985). A scholarly review of the dynamics of violence using the framework developed by Dr. Frantz Fanon, who understood the connections between oppression, mental health, violence, poverty, and colonialism.

Killing Rage: Ending Racism, by Bell Hooks (Owlet, 1996). A searing analysis of racism and its effects. Hooks argues forcefully that self-examination is an important first step toward helping us to find the language of love.

Radio Free Dixie: Robert F. Williams & the Roots of Black Power, by Timothy B. Tyson (The University of North Carolina Press, 1999). A biography of the epic life of Robert F. Williams, President of the Monroe, North Carolina, chapter of the NAACP and a powerful voice for self-defense.

The Open Sore of a Continent: A Personal Narrative of the Nigerian Crisis, by Wole Soyinka (Oxford University Press, 1997). The Nobel Laureate chronicles examples of black-on-black crime in mother Africa.

Soul of a Citizen: Living With Conviction in a Cynical Time, by Paul Rogat Loeb (St. Martins Press, 1999). The author makes the case for social activism as an antidote to despair and surrender.

Life Sentences: Rage and Survival Behind Bars, by Wilbert Rideau and Ron Wikberg (Times Books, 1992). A blistering look at punishment, the death penalty, lost convicts, and the errors of the criminal justice system.

Barbarians to Bureaucrats Corporate Life Cycle Strategies, by Lawrence M. Miller (Fawcett, 1990). A clear and concise view of how companies and corporations grow, and of the kinds of people needed to solve the problems associated with each phase.

The Truly Disadvantaged: The Inner City, the Underclass, and Public Policy, by William Julius Wilson (The University of Chicago Press, 1987). Discusses employment as an essential feature of stable families and how employed men contribute to overall community health.

The Burden of Memory, The Muse of Forgiveness, by Wole Soyinka (Getty Center for Education in the Arts, 2000). Inspired in part by the Truth and Reconciliation Commission in South Africa, Soyinka asks: How can a people go forward if they are not willing to renounce the errors of the past, make amends, and then create a different tomorrow?

Black-On-Black Violence: The Psychodynamics of Black Self-Annihilation in Service of White Domination, by Amos N. Wilson (Afrikan World InfoSystems, 1990). A close examination of the origins of black-on-black violence.

APPENDIX

Work-Related Illnesses

by Peter Davis

Editor's Note: The following material takes up a subject we haven't directly addressed in the text: that certain kinds of work may be hazardous to your health. Ask your doctor if you have questions about symptoms that might match your occupation.

Bird handler: Ornithosis is a disease carried by birds that may be contracted by humans, resulting in a lung infection.

Blacksmith: Infrared light may cause vision problems.

Boot and shoe industry: People in this occupation may be at risk for cancer of the nasal cavity.

Bridge maintenance: The inhalation of spores or fungus may lead to lung infections like pneumonia.

Carpenter/cabinetmaker: Chemicals know as chlorophenols may lead to cancer of the nasal cavity. Hexane (another chemical) may cause inflammation of the nervous system.

Coal miner: Exposure to coal dust may lead to a disease called pneumoconiosis, which is lung disease characterized by emphysema.

Coke iron worker: Coke oven emissions and tar distillates have been associated with cancers of the scrotum and kidney.

Coppersmith: Chemicals used in this industry have been associated with cancers of the lung and trachea.

Copper smelter: Inflammation of the brain, known as toxic encephalitis, may be caused by the use of lead. Symptoms include a stiff neck and mental confusion.

Cotton industry: Byssinosis is a lung disease caused by cotton, flax, hemp, or synthetic dusts.

Cryolite workers: Workers may suffer from discoloration of teeth enamel due to excessive ingestion of fluoride.

Dry cleaners: A chemical called carbon tetrachloride may lead to toxic hepatitis, which is an inflammation of the liver. Symptoms include weakness and yellowing of the eyes or skin (jaundice).

Explosives industry: Certain chemicals used may cause diseases of red blood cells, resulting in fatigue.

Farmer/rancher: Many diseases may be encountered. Some important ones include plague, transmitted by infected fleas; anthrax, transmitted through infected animals and causing open skin lesions; brucellosis, contracted from goats, cattle, pigs, and associated with headaches and malaise; leptospirosis, an infectious disease contracted from dogs, pigs, rodents, or contaminated water that can cause inflammation of the brain.

Fire- and waterproofing: A chemical, ethylene dibromide, had been associated with inflammation of the liver.

Foam and latex manufacturing: Certain chemicals may cause allergies of the skin resulting in hives, or may cause asthma.

Forester/plant worker: Fungus in the soil may cause nodules in the lymph nodes or skin.

Foundry worker: Some chemicals have been associated with cancer of the lung, whereas others may cause inflammation of the brain.

Glassblower: Infrared light may cause vision problems.

Hunter/fur handler: As with the farmer, many diseases may be encountered, usually as a result of coming in contact with infected animals. Some diseases include plague, usually acquired via infected rats and associated with high fever; tularemia, associated with skinning rabbits and causing high fevers; tetanus, in which a toxin causes the neck and jaw muscles to contract; and rabies.

Jewelry maker: Platinum or inorganic mercury may activate a person's asthma.

Leather industry: Copper sulfate may cause a destruction of red blood cells, resulting in fatigue.

Lumberjack: Repetitive body vibration on the job may contribute to Raynaud's phenomenon, or sudden attacks of cold and pain in the fingers or toes.

Medical personnel: Anyone working around sick patients should be aware of the potential exposure to diseases such as tuberculosis and measles, among others.

Metal workers: Chemicals such as mineral-cutting oils have been associated with cancer of the scrotum.

Mining: Silica and talc may be inhaled, which could cause a lung infection (termed silicosis) and result in breathing difficulties.

Nickel smelting: Nickel may be associated with cancer of the nasal cavity. Lead may be used, which can cause inflammation of the brain (and result in headache and mental confusion).

Paper industry: The inhalation of sulfur dioxide may lead to bronchitis.

Petroleum refiners: Soots and tars have been associated with cancer of the scrotum. Exposure to ammonia can cause bronchitis if inhaled in adequate amounts.

Pigment industry: Certain chemicals have been associated with cancer of the bladder and lung. Other chemicals, such as benzene and copper sulfate, may affect the number of blood cells, suppressing the immune system or causing fatigue.

Plant protection: Pesticides and herbicides have been associated with cancer of the lung and bronchus.

Plastics industry: A chemical, trimellitic anhydride, has been associated with asthma, bronchitis, and the destruction of red blood cells, causing fatigue.

Poultry processing: Cumulative trauma, for example, repetitive cutting, may result in inflammation of the nerves in the arms.

Quarryman: Silicon may be inhaled, which could cause a lung infection (termed silicosis) and result in breathing difficulties.

Rayon manufacturer: A chemical, carbon disulfide, has been associated with inflammation of the nervous system.

Refrigeration industry: The inhalation of sulfur dioxide may lead to bronchitis.

Rubber industry: Certain chemicals (benzidine and naphthylamine) have been associated with cancer of the lung and bladder. Workers in this industry may also be at increased risk for leukemia.

Sandblaster: Silica may be inhaled, which could cause a lung infection (termed silicosis) and result in breathing difficulty.

Steel industry: Workers may be at increased risk for lung cancer, but the cause is unknown.

Vinyl chloride industry: Vinyl chloride may contribute to Raynaud's phenomenon, or sudden attacks of cold or pain in the fingers or toes.

Weaver: Anthrax is a disease that may be rapidly fatal.

Welder: Magnesium used in this industry has been associated with cancer of the lung and Parkinson's disease.

Whitewashing industry: A chemical, copper sulfate, has been associated with red blood cell destruction, resulting in fatigue.

INDEX